T0204857

The Weight Loss Triad

2nd Edition

A Comprehensive Guide to Lasting Weight Loss

Dr. Thomas L Halton

Second Edition

Published by Triad Nutrition And Fitness
Glenwood Landing, NY

ISBN 978-0-578-59398-2

The Weight Loss Triad

2nd Edition

Dedication

To my wife, Becky, my son Thomas, and my daughter, Lexi. Without you, this book would have been done at least 3 years sooner! In all seriousness, you guys are the best and mean the world to me.

Table of Contents

Disclaimer

This book is intended for informational and educational purposes only. It is not meant to provide counseling, nor to provide medical advice. Always be sure to consult with your physician before starting any exercise program.

Chapter 1

Introduction To The Weight Loss Triad, 2nd Edition

It is really hard for me to believe that 10 years have passed since I first published *The Weight Loss Triad*. I have to say that I was a bit surprised at how well it did. I never thought I would sell this book to thousands of strangers in just about every state in the U.S.

My original motivation for writing the book was far less ambitious. Successful clients would often ask me if I had my program written down, because they had a friend, relative or coworker out of state that wanted to learn more about it. I figured that this would be a great way to help people who couldn't work with me, so I wrote down my program, self-published it, and figured I'd sell a few dozen copies to my current clients.

Nothing makes me happier than receiving an email or reading an Amazon review from a person I have never met explaining how this book changed their weight, health and life for the better. That type of response is the very reason I do what I do, which is to help people live better lives through positive changes in their diet and exercise program.

After 10 years, I figured it was time to update this book. There are several reasons why I came to this conclusion: 1) There has been a lot of new nutrition and weight loss research in the past 10 years that has influenced my recommendations. While the majority of my program is exactly the same as it was 10 years ago, there have been a few important changes that needed attention. 2) I have had 10 more years of experience working with clients, which has taught me a lot about how to make this program work for people regardless of any obstacles they may be facing. 3) The 1st Edition was written for the general population. I didn't include a lot of the research that guides my recommendations because I didn't want to make things too complicated.

In this edition, I want to let the reader know where they can find the studies that I have used to formulate my recommendations and to provide a summary of this research. This will be very useful to physicians, research PhD's and anyone else that is interested in nutrition and weight loss research. However, I promise not to get too technical or go overboard with the science end of things.

Obesity has reached epidemic proportions in the United States. It is abundantly clear that weight loss is not easy for most people. There are a number of reasons why people have such a hard time losing weight and keeping it off. Reason #1: There is a lot of really bad nutrition information out there that continually pushes people further and further away from research-based evidence. A big part of this is caused by the media. They jump all over a new study, creating powerful headlines with sweeping generalizations designed to sell papers. A few months later they do the same thing with a study that shows the exact opposite. The general population loses confidence in the research process because it looks like scientists are always changing their minds.

Any research scientist of value will tell you that one study does not tell you all that much. You want to see a lot of different types of evidence before making recommendations. One of my professors at Harvard, Dr.

Walter Willett, had a great way of explaining this concept. Think of a nutrition recommendation as a scale. Let's take the relationship between red meat and colon cancer as an example.

Every time a study shows that eating a lot of red meat increases risk of colon cancer, you put a stone on one side of the scale. When a study shows no association, you put a stone on the other side of the scale. If it is a well-designed study with strong internal validity, the stone is a big one. If it is a less well-designed study with some methodological issues, you put a tiny pebble on the scale. Over many years, as studies begin to accumulate, the scale will tip to one side or the other. When it does, that is the time to make a recommendation based on the total accumulation of the evidence.

It is totally normal and appropriate for studies to have conflicting results. It is all part of the scientific process. Studies will vary in their chosen population, dose of nutrient consumed, compliance of the subjects, duration of follow-up, statistical power, measurement and adjustment for confounders, and lots of other things. Differences among these important variables can completely mask associations between dietary exposures and health outcomes. That is why you want to see a whole bunch of studies conducted, and never make or alter recommendations on the results of just one paper. The media doesn't quite understand this, and because they don't, few people in the general population do either.

Another huge source of bad information is nutrition "experts" who have never formally studied nutrition science and don't have the slightest idea of how to read and interpret the research literature. These folks are generally athletes, celebrities, or very attractive men and women who are well spoken and very convincing. The majority of bestselling nutrition and weight loss books are written by these people. They make recommendations based on their opinions and tend to criticize the scientific community if the published research does not agree with these opinions.

I have always found this fascinating. If you had a major tax problem with the IRS, would you not want to consult with a really good accountant who went to an excellent school and is licensed to dispense tax advice? If, God forbid, you were diagnosed with cancer, would you not want to go to a well educated, board certified physician for advice on treatment? If you had a major legal problem, would you not want to hire an ace lawyer who went to one of the best law schools and passed the bar exam? Well, I have news for you: your diet and lifestyle choices can have as much of an impact on your life as any of these other examples, if not more. I have always found it shocking that so many people will take health altering nutrition advice from someone who never studied the subject formally.

The advice I give my clients is based on well-designed research studies. I learned a lot of this research during my doctoral years, conducted some myself, and have read the most influential nutrition research journal every single month since I have graduated (and will for the rest of my life). Rest assured, this program is not opinion based, but research based, as it should be.

The second reason why we struggle with weight loss is our biology. Our body is designed to gain weight quickly and lose it slowly. When I first started studying nutrition and weight loss in the late 1990's, the prevailing theory was that weight loss was simply calories in (your diet) versus calories out (your physical activity). We now know that it is so much more complicated than that.

Our body weight appears to be influenced by a large and continually growing number of factors. Our genes, sleeping patterns, stress levels, blood sugar levels, macronutrient composition, quality of carbohydrates consumed, hormones, visual cues, our brain's addictive response, our level of motivation, what we drink and other factors have all been shown in the research literature to impact our food choices and our weight. We have also learned that once we lose weight, our body fights really hard to put it back on. It does this by increasing hunger and slowing down our metabolism.

The third reason why so many of us struggle with our weight is the current food environment. The wrong foods are everywhere! Think about your food options at an airport, a football game, a movie theater, most restaurants, vending machines, highway rest stops, and coffee shops. Every place you go, there are tons of unhealthy options and very few healthy ones. Add to this the ever-increasing portion sizes of our food and beverages.

I do not mean to paint a bleak picture of your ability to lose weight. You absolutely can! I just want to explain some of the reasons why so many of us have gained weight over the last few decades and why it is so hard to lose it. The solution begins with knowledge. Despite what you may have heard about nutrition research, the process is working. In the last few decades, a ton of well-designed research has been published that helps us understand how our body gains and loses weight. Applying this research will help you to take the steps to lose weight and keep it off. My goal in writing this book is to teach you a bit about the science of weight loss. It may take you some time to apply all you learn, but once you acquire the knowledge, you have the key to your jail cell in the palm of your hand. It is up to you to use it to unlock the door. I can teach you how.

It is important for you to know from the start that this program is not a quick fix. This book is not about following my "revolutionary program" and losing 10 pounds in a week. The sooner you understand this, the sooner you will realize that attaining your weight and health goals will take discipline, sacrifice and time. But the benefits are there. You will be repaid manifold for your effort. I envision this book as being for those who have tried a lot of the "miracle" diets and quick weight loss schemes and now realize that they just don't work. I envision this book being for those who want to know a little about the science of how their body gains and loses weight. I envision this book as being for those who want to know the real truth about how to lose weight safely, effectively and permanently.

It is also important to understand that changes in diet and exercise to lose weight are not temporary solutions that you apply for 3 months and then go back to your old habits. My goal is to help my clients maintain diet and exercise habits for the rest of their lives. A healthy weight and a healthy body require continued effort. If you can't accept this, this is certainly not the book for you. But unfortunately, you better learn to accept this because that is the way it is.

I normally start my first meeting with a new client by telling them a little about myself and my background. Since the format of this book will loosely resemble a consultation with me, here goes.

My name is Thomas L. Halton and I grew up on Long Island, NY. After graduating college and giving law school a try (I lasted one semester-it clearly wasn't the career for me), I realized that a major passion of mine was preventative health. I particularly enjoyed learning about nutrition and exercise science, and then applying what I learned to help people live longer and better lives.

In 1995, I passed the American Council on Exercise Personal Trainer Exam and started working at a gym on Long Island. Shortly thereafter, I founded a small in-home personal training company named Fitness Plus. Almost immediately, the focus of my business became the weight loss client. It did not take me long to realize that this was the job for me; I had truly found my passion. I entered a Masters program in Exercise Science at Queens College in NY to get more formal training in exercise physiology. I was absolutely fascinated to learn the extent that physical activity positively impacts our health. Virtually every system in the human body performs better when we are active and I loved what I was learning and how it could help people.

At this time, I started reading every diet book that I could get my hands on. Back then the popular ones were *The Zone*, *Sugar Busters*, *The Atkins Diet* and *Protein Power*, to name a few. I read them all! I quickly learned that what we eat can have an even bigger impact on our health than being physically active. I decided that I really wanted to learn more about nutrition.

After graduating from my Exercise Science program in 1999, I entered a Masters program in Human Nutrition at the University of Bridgeport, Connecticut. After graduating that program, I sat for the American College of Nutrition Certified Nutrition Specialist examination. This certification, along with my Masters

Degrees and experience would allow me to become a Licensed Nutritionist. I worked full time throughout both of my Masters programs and the combination of the academic knowledge and the more practical knowledge acquired from helping more and more people lose weight became a powerful combination. I wanted to go further with my education.

In 2001, I began my biggest academic challenge to date: I entered Harvard University's doctoral program in Nutritional Epidemiology (the study of how nutrition affects disease). I was very fortunate to be able to study under some of the most gifted nutrition researchers in the world, including Dr. Walter Willett, Dr. Frank Hu and Dr. Frank Sacks. It was at this time that I really started to understand how to interpret the research literature and learned something amazing and also kind of sad: there is a huge and powerful body of nutrition research out there that has much to teach us about how what we eat can impact our long-term health. That is the amazing part. The sad part is that very few people understand how to find this literature and interpret it. Indeed, the field of nutrition is littered with advice that has no basis whatsoever in well-designed research.

I successfully defended my thesis and graduated from Harvard in 2006. Since then, I've opened up 2 additional clinical nutrition counseling and personal training practices, another in Long Island, New York and one in Boston. I have also written 4 books, worked as a research, medical, and corporate consultant, taught Masters and Doctoral students, and worked as a nutrition writer and speaker.

So, what did I learn from all of these degrees, certifications and experience? Well, that is the subject of this book. What you are holding in your hand is everything you need to know in order to lose weight effectively and permanently. At this point in the initial interview, I let the client know that they are about to receive an overwhelming amount of information. Most of which will require serious lifestyle changes that are not easy at first. I tell them that I am about to explain everything that they can do to lose weight the fastest, healthiest and most permanent way.

I don't expect them to immediately follow every principle perfectly. That is not really possible. I also tell them that I'm giving them the gold standard and that they will still lose weight with the silver or bronze standard, just a bit more slowly.

I have had a few rare clients that were able to incorporate just about everything right away, and let me say, they get amazing results. Most of my successful clients, however, focused on one area at a time. In the first few weeks they worked on resistance training and then focused on cardiovascular exercise and finally diet and lifestyle issues. This took place over a period of weeks and/or months. I think this is a great way to break down the program into smaller pieces that are easier to focus on.

Losing weight is a very personal thing and everyone has their own strengths and weaknesses that will influence their progress. Furthermore, the path to weight loss is rarely a straight line. There are peaks and valleys. There will be times that you feel it's a snap and the pounds are rolling off. Then there will be times when the scale doesn't budge or you've relapsed a bit and the situation seems hopeless. This is all normal; expect it, but know this- I have never met a person in all of my years that wasn't able to lose weight with these changes. Everyone who follows these guidelines can make significant and permanent positive changes to their bodies.

I guess now would be a good time to explain the major concept and the name of this book: The Weight Loss Triad. A triad is simply a group of 3. Three is a very important number for those of you trying to lose weight. Three is the number of areas that need attention if your goal is permanent weight loss. More specifically, the three areas are: 1) Diet, 2) Cardiovascular exercise and 3) Resistance training.

The goal of the dietary component is to ensure a stable blood sugar. Humans were designed to have a stable blood sugar and most of the foods put on this Earth for us promote blood sugar stability. However, we have changed our food supply by processing and refining foods to the point that they barely resemble the foods we were intended to eat. Getting back to a stable blood sugar will decrease cravings and set your body up for fat burning instead of fat storage.

The goal of the cardiovascular exercise program is, quite simply, to burn calories. Obviously, this will help reduce stores of body fat. The goal of the resistance training program is two-fold. As we age, we start to lose muscle. Muscle is a metabolically active tissue, it takes a lot of calories to maintain muscle. The first goal of the weight training component is to not only stop this loss of lean tissue, but to add to it so you burn more calories every day, just by breathing!

The second reason to include resistance training during weight loss has to do with the human body defense mechanism to hold on to body fat. When you lose weight, your body gets nervous and wants to protect fat reserves for the future. Therefore, it will give up a bit of fat but after a point will start to burn muscle in addition to fat. So, a person goes on a commercial weight loss plan and loses 10 pounds without resistance training. Little do they know that some of that weight loss was fat but a significant amount was muscle. A pound of muscle burns three times as many calories as a pound of fat. So, muscle tissue that was previously burning calories each and every day is now ancient history.

Because of this drop in metabolism, the dieter hits a brick wall and stops losing weight. Since they are no longer losing weight, they stop their diet and begin to eat as they used to. They quickly gain back the 10 lbs. they lost plus more because their metabolism is now operating with less muscle. This sequence is often repeated several times and is largely responsible for the yo-yo dieting syndrome that impacts so many of us. Resistance training helps to lessen this breakdown of muscle with weight loss so more of the weight you lose will be fat. This results in permanent weight loss instead of yo-yo dieting.

It is easy to think of these 3 areas as a pyramid.

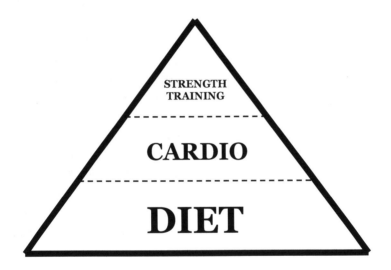

You may be familiar with the USDA Food Guide Pyramid or the Mediterranean Diet Pyramid. This weight loss pyramid is based on a similar principle. The most important part is the base; in this case diet. The next most important part is cardiovascular exercise and the third most important aspect of the program is resistance or strength training. This is a simple and quick way to show you how you should prioritize the different components of this program. In my experience, for those trying to lose weight, 50% of their results will come from dietary change, 30% from the cardiovascular exercise component and 20% from resistance training. Having said this, all three components are necessary to maximize fat loss. The pyramid is a rough guide to let you know how you should prioritize your valuable time and energy.

It is also important to realize that there is not just one way to lose weight. There are people that are successful using low fat diets, low carb diets, Paleo diets, high protein diets, etc. However, you need to realize that weight loss does not occur in a vacuum. You need to consider how your choice of weight loss strategy will impact the rest of your life, including your quality of life and long-term risk of chronic disease.

It is certainly not ideal to choose a diet that helps you lose weight, but because of what you are eating (or avoiding) you increase your risk of chronic disease, like heart disease, diabetes or cancer. Similarly, if your diet helps you lose weight, but you are starving all the time and miserable, that is not good either. My plan keeps this big picture in mind.

After all of my years of research and education, there are several reasons why I recommend this strategy. The first is that you will not be hungry on this plan. When your blood sugar is stable, hunger and food cravings both decrease dramatically. This makes it much easier to stay on the program long-term.

The second reason is that all of my recommendations are based on what the latest research tells us about the relationship between our diet and our risk of chronic disease, such as heart disease, stroke, diabetes, cancer and Alzheimer's disease. I won't recommend something in your diet or exercise plan that may enhance weight loss, but potentially harms you in some other way. The health and quality of life of my clients are my biggest priorities. That is why I think this program is so great. It not only helps you lose weight, but will reduce your risk of chronic disease and knocks out your hunger and food cravings. Talk about a win, win, win!

One last thing I want to cover before we really get started. I want you to enjoy your life. Eating the wrong food sometimes is part of that. There are certain scenarios in your life where eating perfectly healthy isn't going to happen, and that is totally OK. My two favorite sports teams are the New York Jets and the New York Islanders. I am illogically obsessed with both of them. I go to a lot of Jets and Islanders games. Going to these games is one of the most fun things that I do with my kids, my wife, and my friends. I am not going to eat a can of black beans with a side of cashews, an apple with a bottle of water at these games. I am going to eat fun, delicious junk food along with my family and friends. The food is a big part of the fun for me.

My wife and I were at a wedding a couple of years ago. An old friend of mine was getting married at a beautiful golf course on the North Shore of Long Island. We sat at a table with a couple of acquaintances and a bunch of strangers. They were all really nice. When dinner came, one of the women at our table politely declined her plate, reached into a bag and took out a Tupperware container with a broiled chicken breast, steamed vegetables, and rice. She bought her food with her to the wedding. While a part of me admired her discipline and dedication to her diet, another part of me thought it was a little nuts. To me, worrying about your diet that much takes away a lot of fun out of your life. The food at the wedding, by the way, was awesome!

Now don't get me wrong, eating healthy is a major focus for me and helping others eat healthy is one of my biggest passions. But I've got some good news for you. You don't have to be 100% on this program. There are times you are totally allowed to go off the plan and eat something delicious that you are not supposed to. However, you will do so in a planned and controlled manner.

There are 3 reasons why this is not only OK, but I insist upon it: #1) You don't have to be 100% on your diet to attain all of your weight loss and health goals; 85-90% adherence will absolutely get the job done. #2) Going off your diet a couple of times a week promotes long term adherence. For example, a big part of the program is to limit refined grains like white bread. If I told you that you can never have a slice of pizza again in your life, half of you would laugh at me and throw away the book. The other half may try it for a couple of weeks and realize it just is not realistic. However, if you are allowed to have your favorite foods a couple of times a week, it is much more realistic to stay on this plan long term. #3) We can't always control our food. We get invited to weddings, dinner parties, business dinners, etc. We don't always get to pick our food at these events. Having a few meals per week that you can eat anything makes navigating these events a snap. At the end of the day, it is important to learn that there is a time to eat for fun (some of the time) and a time to eat for health (most of the time). I once read somewhere that food is medicine that you take 3 times per day. I honestly can't remember who wrote it, but truer words have never been written!

In the remainder of this book, I'll take you through each of the three components of the program in detail. In Chapters 2-6 we will focus on your diet. Chapter 7 is all about cardio. Chapters 8 and 9 cover resistance training. Chapters 10 and 11 will cover material that will make this plan a whole lot easier to fit into your life, including frequently asked questions, lifestyle factors and some important tips to help you stay focused. I will also end each chapter with some action steps to help you focus on applying what you have learned. My goal is teach you everything that I know in order to help you attain your weight loss goals in a safe and efficient manner. Along the way we'll accomplish other goals that may or not be important to you, such as increasing your energy, reducing the effects of stress, improving your sleeping habits, reducing the risk of heart disease, stroke, diabetes and cancer, boosting your immune system, decreasing the risk of osteoporosis, decreasing symptoms of anxiety and depression and boosting that all important self-confidence. When I start with a new client, I really feel as though we are going on a mission together. There will be ups and downs, good times and bad, but the goal is attainable. My job is to light a flame under you until it catches. Because once you realize the benefits of living the way I'm about to show you, you'll never want to go back. Are you ready? Are you psyched? Let's get to it.

<u>ACTION STEPS FOR THIS CHAPTER</u>

1. Realize mentally that weight loss is not quick or easy.
2. Realize that changes in diet and exercise habits need to be permanent for weight loss to be permanent.
3. Pace yourself with the lifestyle changes you will soon learn. Don't expect to change everything overnight. Chip away at it and try to get a little better each week. We are looking for progress, not perfection.
4. Understand that when it comes to weight loss, 50% of your results will come from your dietary changes, 30% from your cardiovascular exercise habits and 20% from your resistance training program. Prioritize accordingly.

Chapter 2

Introduction To The Dietary Plan;
50% Of Weight Loss Success

As mentioned previously, your diet is the most important component of your weight loss program and will have the biggest impact on your success or failure. So, now it's time to find out how to eat for success! The foods we eat can be broken down into 3 basic categories called macronutrients; they are protein, fat and carbohydrate. Although most foods contain all 3 of these macronutrients, one is usually represented much more than the others. In this section of the book, I will briefly explain the function of each of these macronutrients and provide guidance on how to choose the best foods to help you lose weight and improve your health. At the end, we'll put it all together. I'll show you sample meal plans that will help you tailor this way of eating to your own personal preferences.

Now would be a good time to describe my own personal nutrition philosophy. I guess I am what you'd call an "evolutionary" nutritionist. I believe that Mother Nature knows a lot more about what we should be eating than anyone or anything else. Certain foods were put on this Earth for us to consume while our internal systems were evolving. Man came along and started refining and processing foods and messed up this general formula for good health. If you take a look at the diet of the typical

American, the vast majority of foods consumed are no longer in their natural form. Fitness trailblazer Jack LaLane was once asked about what constitutes a healthy diet and he responded, "If man made it, don't eat it". In many ways, this is a pretty efficient answer to just about every single nutrition question ever asked.

A major problem with the processed food that we eat today has to do with how it impacts our blood sugar. The foods put on this Earth for us to consume, for the most part, have a very easy effect on our blood sugar. When we eat them, our blood glucose level rises gradually and we release a small amount of insulin to lower it back down. This is the way it should be. In fact, for 99% of the time that humans have existed, this is exactly how we have eaten. When we eat processed, refined carbo-hydrates, our blood glucose levels rise sharply and we need to release a very large amount of insulin to handle this peak. As we will learn shortly, this is a big problem. In the past 50 or so years, we have dramatically in-creased our consumption of refined carbohydrate foods in this country. It is not a coincidence that our rates of obesity have skyrocketed during this time.

The glycemic index (GI for short) is a measure of how much a carbohydrate containing food increases your blood sugar. Pure glucose is the reference for this measure and has a glycemic index of 100. White bread has a GI of 71, white rice has a GI of 75 and a baked potato has a GI of 94 (1). These all fall into the category of high glycemic index carbohydrates. On the other hand, an apple has a GI of 40, lentils have a GI of 22 and peas have a GI of 39 (1). These carbs all have a much easier impact on your blood sugar.

There is also a measure called the insulin index (II for short). This is a measure of how high your insulin rises after consuming a carbohydrate containing food. White bread has an II of 100, white rice has an II of 79, cookies have an II of 92 and potatoes have an II of 121 (2). In comparison, lentils have an II of 58 and corn has an II of 53 (2). The glycemic and insulin indices show us that all carbohydrates do not have the same impact on our body, even when they are consumed in equal amounts.

Choosing the wrong type of carbs is where we run into problems. Large swings in blood sugar and insulin levels have a variety of negative effects. For starters, high insulin levels drive blood glucose below baseline and cause an increase in hunger. This is backed up by solid research.

Dr. David Ludwig, who is a professor at Harvard Medical School and a leading researcher on glycemic index and obesity, published a review on the role of GI on the obesity epidemic. In this paper, Dr. Ludwig presents 16 studies that tested high glycemic meals vs. low glycemic meals. In 15 of the 16 studies reviewed, a low glycemic test meal resulted in greater satiety, decreased hunger or decreased subsequent energy intake when compared to a high glycemic meal (3).

Here is a more detailed look at one of these studies: 12 overweight men consumed two different meals on two separate occasions and then had several measurements taken (4). Both meals used similar recipes and had the exact same number of calories. The key difference was that certain ingredients were altered to make the meal high glycemic index or low glycemic index. One meal had a GI of 84 and the other had a GI of 37.

Two hours after the high GI meal, plasma glucose was 2.4 times higher than after the low GI meal. Four hours after the high GI meal, glucose levels were significantly lower and hunger was significantly higher when compared to the low GI meal. Another really interesting finding in this study is that after the high GI meal, an area of the brain associated with reward and cravings was stimulated. This was not seen after the low GI meal and suggests that there may be an addictive component to high glycemic carbohydrate consumption.

Can these swings in blood sugar and insulin increase rate of weight gain? The research suggests that they can. Higher insulin levels promote fat storage and inhibit lipoprotein lipase, an enzyme that tells your body to burn fat (5). High secretion of insulin has been also independently associated with weight gain (6).

In a study of more than 120,000 men and women conducted by the Harvard School of Public Health, researchers found that many of the foods associated with long-term weight gain had a high glycemic index (7). This list included refined grains, sweets and desserts, sugar sweetened beverages, potatoes, French fries and potato chips. It is no surprise that many of the foods that were significantly associated with weight loss were low glycemic, including fruits, vegetables and whole grains.

This combination of increased hunger and enhanced fat deposition that occurs when eating the wrong type of carbohydrate is a major concern for those looking to lose weight. The good news is that stabilizing these dramatic highs and lows in your blood sugar can be prevented, and quite easily.

There are basically 2 strategies to ensure a stable blood sugar. 1) Choose carbohydrates that are easy on the blood sugar. 2) Every time you eat, combine a fat containing food, a protein containing food and a carbohydrate containing food. The addition of fat and protein to a carbohydrate slows the entry of that carbohydrate into the blood stream.

The human body contains macronutrient specific digestive enzymes. There are enzymes that just digest fat, enzymes that just digest protein and enzymes that just digest carbohydrate. For example, when you eat a plain bagel for breakfast, the carbohydrate digesting enzymes have direct access to the carbohydrate and convert it to blood sugar at a very fast rate, causing a spike in blood glucose. Now, if you ate that same bagel with some lox (protein) and cream cheese (fat), the protein, fat and carbohydrate would mix up in your stomach. The carbohydrate digesting enzymes would have to work around the fat and protein, which takes time, and therefore the carbohydrate would be digested much more slowly, resulting in a lower peak glucose and insulin level.

The research literature shows that adding a source of fat (8) or a source of protein (9) to a carbohydrate significantly reduces the post prandial glucose response. Adding both appears to have a synergistic effect. In an interesting study, 12 subjects were given 5 test meals before having their glucose measured (10); white rice, white rice with vegetables, white rice with chicken, white rice with oil and finally white rice with chicken, vegetables and oil.

When the white rice was eaten alone, the measured GI was 96. Adding a vegetable dropped the measured GI to 82. Adding the chicken (a protein) to the white rice lowered the measured GI to 73. Adding the oil (a fat) to the white rice lowered the measured GI to 68. When the vegetable, chicken, and oil were added to the white rice, the measured GI dropped all the way to 50.

Probably the most important thing to remember about this plan is the following: Make sure you include some protein, some fat and some low glycemic carbohydrate at every meal. This is pivotal to maintaining a steady blood sugar. We'll get into the details in the next few chapters but for now just try to grasp this concept.

In the next part of our journey, we'll go through each of these three macronutrients, learn a bit about their functions and then find out which to focus on and which to avoid. We'll list the best choices for fat, protein and carbohydrate and then every time you eat, you will simply pick one food from the carbohydrate list, one from the fat list and one from the protein list. We'll then get into some meal planning and portions sizes and then you'll be good to go on diet.

<u>ACTION STEPS FOR THIS CHAPTER</u>

1. Realize that stabilizing your blood sugar is absolutely critical to weight loss success.
2. Realize that not all carbohydrates effect our body in the same manner. Some have an easy impact on our blood sugar, some cause a massive spike in our blood sugar.
3. In order to stabilize your blood sugar and set the stage for weight loss, combine a low glycemic carbohydrate with a healthy source of fat and protein at each and every meal.

Chapter 3

How to Pick the Right Protein

Protein is a great macronutrient to start with because most people already know what foods are high in protein and almost all of these foods are permitted. Eating enough protein is of paramount importance to the maintenance of optimal health. Aside from water, protein forms the major portion of a lean human body, just about 16 percent of body weight.

Some of the major functions of protein include:

1. The formation of vital body compounds. Each and every cell contains protein. All of the following are made primarily of protein: muscle, enzymes, lipoproteins, connective tissue, clotting factors, immune factors, a wide variety of hormones as well as the supporting structure inside bones. Most of these vital components are in a constant state of breakdown, reconstruction and repair. If a person doesn't eat enough protein, over many weeks and months, the protein repairing and rebuilding slows down. Eventually skeletal muscle, the heart, the liver and other organs will decrease in size or amount to compensate; only your brain will resist this breakdown.
2. Maintaining acid/base balance.
3. Ensuring fluid balance.

4. <u>Immune function.</u> Proteins contribute vital parts of the cells used by the immune system.
5. <u>Protein can provide the body with a ready source of energy.</u> In general, protein contributes less than 5% of the body's total energy need.
6. <u>Formation of glucose.</u> During times of inadequate carbohydrate intake, our body has the ability to make glucose, a major cellular fuel, out of amino acids from proteins.

Now here is the take home message of this chapter: *MAKE SURE YOU EAT SOME PROTEIN AT EVERY SINGLE MEAL.* Protein slows the entry of carbohydrate into your blood stream. Remember, the fundamental philosophy behind this style of eating is the maintenance of a steady blood sugar, as nature intended. The inclusion of protein with every meal can help you maintain this steady blood sugar as well as provide a number of other benefits.

For example, there is evidence that those who consume higher amounts of protein at a meal have a greater sense of fullness (1,2) and tend to eat fewer calories at subsequent meals (3,4). I have found this to be quite true with my clients. There is also strong evidence that protein has a higher thermic effect than fat or carbohydrate (5). The thermic effect of food is the increase in energy expenditure above baseline following consumption. This energy is required for digestion, absorption and disposal of ingested nutrients. Therefore, in order for your body to break down and use the protein you eat, you have to burn more calories than you do for fat or carbohydrates. While this difference is relatively small, these extra calories do add up over weeks and months.

The A to Z Weight Loss Study is a well-designed randomized trial that examined the efficacy of 4 popular diets in over 300 overweight women; The Ornish Diet (very low fat), The LEARN Diet (a standard low-fat diet), The Zone Diet (40% carb, 30% fat, 30% protein) and The Atkins Diet (low carb) (14). After one year of follow-up, women on the Atkins diet lost significantly more weight than women in the other groups. The researchers believed that the higher protein content of the Atkins diet was a big reason for the difference.

Types Of Protein And Your Health

Protein on its own does not seem to have a major impact on risk of chronic disease. However, what comes along with the protein you consume can in a big way. When your protein is packaged with sodium, saturated fat and industrial processing ingredients, you can run into trouble. On the other hand, when your protein is packaged with fiber, omega 3 fatty acids, vitamins, minerals or plant phytochemicals, it can have a power-fully positive impact on your health. The research literature backs this up.

Let's start with some of the less healthy sources of protein. A high consumption of red meat has been associated with an increased risk of heart disease (6), all-cause mortality (7), type 2 diabetes (8), and cancer (7). In a 2015 review of over 800 studies, the World Health Organization's International Agency for Research on Cancer classified red meat as "probably carcinogenic to humans" (9).

Processed red meat, such as bacon, sausage, pepperoni, hot dogs, and salami, has often shown even stronger associations with disease outcomes than red meat in the research literature. Processed red meat has been associated with an increased risk of heart disease (6), all-cause mortality (7), type 2 diabetes (8), and cancer (7). The International Agency for Research on Cancer classified processed red meat as "carcinogenic to humans" (9).

It is a really good idea to strictly limit red meat and processed meats. You don't have to totally avoid them, but you don't want to make them your go to protein choice. Having a steak or a burger once a week or so probably won't do you much harm, but I would not go much higher than that.

One of the most impressive studies that I ever read on protein and risk of disease was published in 2012 in the journal *Archives of Internal Medicine* (2). In this investigation, 37,698 men from Harvard's Health Professional Follow-up Study and 83,644 women from Harvard's Nurses' Health Study were followed for over 20 years. In these subjects, substituting one serving per day of fish, poultry, legumes or low-fat dairy for one serving of red meat or processed red meat was associated with a significantly reduced risk of death from any cause. Focusing on these leaner sources of protein is definitely the way to go.

The OmniHeart Study is a well-designed randomized trial that was published in the *Journal of the American Medical Association* in 2005 (10). In this investigation, 164 men and women consumed three different diets for 6 weeks each. The first diet was a high carbohydrate diet (15% protein, 58% carbohydrate, 27% fat). The second diet was a high unsaturated fat diet (15% protein, 48% carbohydrate, 37% fat). The third diet was high in protein (25% protein, 48% carbohydrate, 27% fat).

Compared to the high carbohydrate diet, the high protein diet significantly reduced systolic blood pressure, diastolic blood pressure, total cholesterol, LDL cholesterol and triglycerides. These are all very important risk factors for cardiovascular disease.

During my doctoral years at Harvard, my research group conducted a couple of very interesting studies on the health effects of low carbohydrate diets. We found that women following a low carb diet who picked healthy, vegetable sources of fat and protein had a 30% lower risk of heart disease over 20 years when compared to women consuming a low-fat, high carbohydrate diet (11). This benefit was not seen in women who chose less healthy animal sources of protein and fat. We found very similar results when looking at risk of type 2 diabetes (12).

So, the research does point to the idea that increasing your protein a bit is not only safe, but comes along with substantial health benefits, as long as you are picking healthy sources of protein. Having said that, if you have certain medical conditions, particularly those influencing the kidneys, you will want to check with your doctor before increasing your level of protein intake.

There is one other important thing to mention: there is some limited evidence that a very high protein intake may be associated with an increased risk of bone fracture. The theory here is that a lot of protein increases the need for calcium in order to buffer the acids that form with a higher protein diet. In the Nurses' Health Study, women consuming the highest amount of protein (95 grams per day) had a 22% increased risk of forearm fracture when compared to women consuming the least protein. (68 grams per day) (13). Hip fracture was not associated with protein consumption in this investigation.

Guidelines For Protein Consumption

Currently in the United States, we consume about 15% of our calories as protein. Raising the percent of protein from 15% to 20-25% is a good idea for those trying to lose weight, particularly if that additional 5-10% increase in protein comes at the expense of refined carbohydrate. I also feel that this is a safe level of protein intake for healthy individuals.

Good Protein Choices

Lean Meats: Chicken and turkey without the skin are good choices. Lean cuts of red meat such as filet mignon, pork tenderloin, roast beef or 93% lean ground beef can be consumed occasionally. I usually recommend a serving or two a week max for the lean red meats.

Seafood: Any type of fish or shell fish are permitted. Shoot for 3 to 4 servings of seafood per week. This balances the healthy aspects of seafood (good source of protein and omega-3 fatty acids) and limits the potential problems (PCP and mercury contamination). Please see additional information on seafood in the *A Note About Fish* section in just a few pages.

Low Fat Dairy: Skim milk, low-fat cottage cheese, fat free plain yogurt and low-fat cheese are all good choices here. See *A Note About Dairy* below for a discussion on how often you should consume dairy.

Eggs: Eggs are a very good source of protein. Egg whites can be consumed as often as you like. Shoot for no more than 6 egg yolks per week due to their high cholesterol content.

Legumes: Legumes are a nutrition powerhouse and a great source of vegetable protein. Good choices here include black beans, pink beans, navy beans, chick peas, lentils and hummus. The research on the health effects of soy protein tends to go back and forth a bit, so I would limit consumption to a few servings per week.

Protein Choices To Strictly Limit
Fatty Cuts Of Red Meat: Hamburger, pork and fatty cuts of steak are high in saturated fat and when cooked can form harmful substances called nitrosamines that have been associated with an increased risk of cancer.

Processed Meats: Hot dogs, sausages, bacon, pepperoni, bologna, ham, salami, pastrami and other fatty deli meats should be strictly limited. They are high in saturated fat and contain nitrates and other processing agents that have been associated with an increased risk of heart disease and cancer.

Full Fat Dairy: Whole milk, full fat yogurt, full fat cottage cheese and whole cheeses should be strictly limited. These are very high in saturated fat, which has been associated with an increased risk of heart disease.

A Note About Dairy

There has been some recent controversy concerning the importance of dairy products in our diet. A lot of nutritionists recommend dairy as a source of both protein and calcium. I have some serious questions about whether this is such a good idea. To start with, I always view the diet from an evolutionary standpoint. In other words, what foods were put on this earth for man and woman to consume? Were we really meant to consume large amounts of dairy products?

Our digestive systems evolved over 100's and 1000's of years on the foods that were put here for us by Mother Nature, God or whatever you are comfortable with. If you take a look at nature, no animals consume milk after the age of about 6 months to a year and no animal drinks another species' milk; ever! So, I have my doubts about the large number of servings of dairy recommended by the U.S. Department of Agriculture's MyPlate.

Ironically, diary may not even be good at the one thing that everyone is consuming it for; strengthening bones. In a meta-analysis of 12 studies, there was no association between dietary calcium consumption and risk of hip fracture (15). In this study, men and women who consumed over 1,110 mg of calcium per day had no lower risk of hip fracture than those consuming about 400 mg per day. And this wasn't just 1 study, it was a summary of 12 studies. Furthermore, there is some evidence that a high dairy consumption may even be harmful. A high calcium and dairy consumption have been associated with an increased risk of prostate cancer (16) and ovarian cancer (17).

I am not saying that calcium is not an important part of our diet, it totally is. I am just saying we don't need as much of it as most people think and we certainly don't need to drink tons and tons of milk every day. I would probably say it is fine to have one serving of dairy most days of the week, but not much more than that. One serving of dairy plus the calcium you get if you are consuming a healthy diet is more than adequate.

Remember, physical activity is one of the very best ways to prevent osteoporosis. On this program you'll get plenty of that, trust me!

A Note About Fish

Fish are an excellent source of protein and omega 3 fatty acids, which for years have been shown to have a multitude of health benefits in the research literature. You may have been reading in the paper about mercury toxicity in our fish supply. This is a legitimate concern, particularly for women who are pregnant or trying to become pregnant. While mercury toxicity can cause a variety of symptoms in humans, it is particularly harmful to developing fetuses. Specifically, it can cause a decreased neurological development.

Mercury from industry and other sources accumulates in the tissue of fish dwelling in polluted regions. The larger and more predatory fish tend to accumulate the highest levels and should be avoided by pregnant women, women who are trying to become pregnant, nursing mothers, and small children. They are: Swordfish, Shark, King Mackerel, Tilefish, Orange Roughy, Marlin and Albacore-, Bigeye- or Yellow-fin Tuna.

Sometimes, pregnant women want to play it safe and avoid seafood altogether in an effort to protect their baby. This is a very bad idea. Omega 3 fatty acids from seafood are essential for the proper brain development of the fetus. If you are pregnant, trying to become pregnant, or nursing, talk to your doctor about the right type and amount of seafood you should be consuming. For the rest of us, 3 servings of seafood a week is right where you want to be. Let your tastes guide you, but I would recommend also limiting consumption of the high mercury fish species (Swordfish, Shark, King Mackerel, Tilefish, Orange Roughy, Marlin and Albacore-, Bigeye- or Yellow-fin Tuna).

ACTION STEPS FOR THIS CHAPTER

1. Protein helps to stabilize blood sugar, increase satiety and decrease subsequent energy intake. Make sure to include a healthy source of protein each time you eat. Shoot for roughly 20% of calories as protein.
2. Depending on what comes along with it, your choice of protein can have a powerfully positive or negative impact on your risk of chronic disease.
3. Focus on lean meats, seafood, legumes and low-fat dairy products.
4. Strictly limit red meat, processed meats like bacon, sausage and hot dogs and high fat dairy products.

Chapter 4

How To Pick Healthy Fats

Fat is without a doubt the most misunderstood nutrient in the field of nutrition. Fats, also known as lipids, are a wide variety of compounds that share one common trait; they do not dissolve readily in water. Triglycerides are the most common form of fat found in food as well as the human body. A triglyceride consists of a glycerol with three fatty acids. Lipids that are solid at room temperature, like butter, are called fats. Lipids that are liquid at room temperature, like olive oil, are called oils. Some of the major functions of fat include:

1. Providing energy for the body.
2. Storing energy for the body.
3. Insulating and protecting vital organs.
4. Transportation of the fat-soluble vitamins (A, D, E and K).

Fat has gotten a very bad reputation. Early nutrition research suggested that certain fats were associated with an increased risk of heart disease and cancer. Another knock against fat is that it is very calorie dense, providing 9 calories per gram as compared to protein and carbohydrate, which provide 4 calories per gram. For these reasons, the main thrust of nutrition advice in the 1980's and 1990's was to drastically reduce the amount of fat in our diets. The motivating force behind this advice was to prevent disease and decrease the incidence of obesity.

However, making such blanket recommendations concerning dietary fat was akin to throwing out the baby with the bath water. Let's start with the weight gain issue. It was assumed that the higher intakes of dietary fat were related to obesity. Not necessarily. In this country, the percent of fat in our diet has slowly dropped from 40% to 34% of calories over the past few decades. In this time, the rates of obesity have skyrocketed. While there are other important factors at play such as physical activity and total calories consumed, this statistic certainly doesn't support the theory that decreasing the percentage of fat in the diet will have a major effect on weight loss.

At the end of the day, there is really no evidence that the percentage of fat in your diet influences your body weight. This is very likely a surprise to most people. I do admit that the amount of fat needs to be monitored in the diet, but in my years of clinical experience and research, I am not at all convinced that a low-fat diet is the path to permanent weight loss or greater health.

On to disease risk. As we will shortly learn, some fats are good for you and others, not so much. Because this is true, you really only need to limit certain types of dietary fat. Let's get this straightened out! There are four types of fat in our diets. Three of these are natural and one is man-made. It is imperative that you get to know these well.

Trans Fat

Let's start with the man-made fat: partially hydrogenated vegetable oil or trans fat. Trans fat is produced through the commercial hydrogenation of polyunsaturated oils (plant oils). Hydrogen is bubbled through the oil at a certain pressure and in the presence of a nickel catalyst. This changes the chemical structure of the fat. What this means for us is that our body has to deal with an unnatural fat that is incorporated into our cell structures and membranes.

There are a variety of reasons why manufacturers have traditionally used hydrogenated oils in food products:

1. Hydrogenation removes essential fatty acids such as linoleic and alpha linolenic acid. These fatty acids tend to oxidize over time, which can turn the fat rancid. Therefore, a big reason for the use of hydrogenated oils is to prolong shelf life.

2. Hydrogenation increases the melting point of oil so that the product is solid at 25° Celsius. This acts to improve the texture and consistency of many commercially prepared foods.

3. Using this type of oil is cheaper for the manufacturers.

Believe it or not, some trans fats are found in nature. A tiny percent of dairy fat is trans. However, this amount is generally considered too small to produce significant negative health effects. In years past, commercially prepared oils found in fried and baked food and margarines were a huge source of trans fat in our diets.

After a great deal of lobbying by consumer advocate groups, in 2006 trans fats were required to appear on food labels. This was great news. Because trans fats were known to be unhealthy, the requirement of listing them on food labels has influenced manufacturers to eliminate them from their products. After all, they don't want their product to be perceived as unhealthy.

The FDA went even further in 2015 when it ruled that partially hydrogenated vegetable oil, the major source of dietary trans fat, is no longer "generally recognized as safe". Food companies were given until 2018 to eliminate trans fats from their food products. This is a major public health victory and the combination of education, food labeling and the FDA ruling have dramatically reduced trans fat consumption in the U.S. In one study using data from the National Health and Nutrition Examination Survey, blood levels of trans fat decreased 58% between 2000 and 2009 (1).

Saturated Fat

Saturated fats are fats that contain no double bonds. All of the carbons are saturated with hydrogen. They are mostly found in animal products. Sources of saturated fat include: fatty cuts of steak and other red meat, butter, full fat dairy products like whole milk, ice cream, cheese and whole yogurt. Bacon and fatty cold cuts are also high in saturated fat.

Monounsaturated Fat

Monounsaturated fats have a slightly different structure than other fats. They contain one double bond and therefore, not all of their carbons are saturated with hydrogen. You'll find these types of fatty acids in olive oil and canola oil, as well as a variety of nuts and avocados.

Polyunsaturated Fat

These fats are similar to monounsaturated fats but instead of having just one double bond, they have two or more. These fats are found in most nuts and plant oils like corn oil, soybean oil and safflower oil.

Health Affects Of Dietary Fats

Mortality

In probably the most comprehensive cohort study ever conducted on the subject of dietary fat and risk of death, 83,349 women from the Nurses' Health Study and 42,884 men from the Health Professional Follow-up Study were followed for over 25 years (2). Subjects who consumed the most saturated fat and trans fat had a significantly higher risk of death when compared to subjects that consumed the lowest amount of saturated fat and trans fat. Subjects who consumed the most mono- and polyunsaturated fat had a significantly lower risk of death when compared to subjects who consumed the lowest amount of these fats. Let's break this down by looking at the impact of these fats on individual diseases.

Heart Disease

Each of the four types of fats was examined for their association with heart disease in over 80,000 women from the Nurses' Health Study (3). After 14 years of follow-up, there were 939 cases of fatal heart disease and non-fatal myocardial infarction. Following are some of the major findings of this important paper:

- Each increase of 5% of energy as saturated fat was associated with a 17% increased risk of heart disease as compared to a 5% increase in carbohydrates.

- A 2% increase in energy as trans fat was associated with a 93% increased risk of heart disease compared to equivalent energy from carbohydrate.
- A 5% increase in energy from mono-unsaturated fat was associated with a 19% decreased risk of heart disease.
- A 5% increase in energy from polyunsaturated fat was associated with a 38% decreased risk of coronary heart disease.
- Total fat was not associated with risk of heart disease.

Several randomized trials back-up these findings. The PREDIMED investigation randomly assigned 7,447 subjects to one of 3 diets: a Mediterranean diet high in olive oil, a Mediterranean diet high in mixed nuts or a low-fat control diet (4). The primary endpoint was major cardiovascular events, which included myocardial infarction, stroke or death from cardiovascular causes. The trial was actually stopped after less than 5 years because the subjects on the Mediterranean diet were doing so much better than the low-fat group.

The Mediterranean group supplemented with olive oil had a 30% lower risk of having a major cardiovascular event and the Mediterranean group supplemented with mixed nuts had a 28% lower risk when compared to the low-fat control group. The researchers credit most of the benefit to the increased monounsaturated and polyunsaturated fats consumed by subjects in the Mediterranean diet groups.

In the OmniHeart Randomized Trial, 164 hypertensive adults were put on a high carbohydrate, high protein, or high fat diet (mostly monounsaturated fat) for a period of 6 weeks (5). Compared to the high carbohydrate diet, the high fat diet significantly reduced blood pressure and triglycerides and significantly raised HDL cholesterol.

In the Lyon Diet Heart Study, 605 heart attack survivors were randomized to either a low-fat diet or a Mediterranean diet high in olive oil and omega-3 fats (6). The trial was stopped after only two and a half years because the benefit of the Mediterranean diet was so strong. Compared to the low-fat diet group, the Mediterranean group had a 70% reduction in new heart attacks or death from any cause.

The ratio of total cholesterol to HDL cholesterol is an important indicator of one's risk of developing heart disease. The lower this ratio is, the lower your risk of heart disease. In a meta-analysis of 60 randomized controlled trials, this ratio significantly decreased when saturated fats were replaced by unsaturated fats (7). This study also showed that when saturated fats were replaced by carbohydrates, the ratio of total cholesterol to HDL cholesterol did not significantly change. Furthermore, when carbohydrates replaced fats in the diet, triglycerides increased. Higher triglycerides are associated with an increased risk of heart disease.

Type 2 Diabetes

Your choice of dietary fats can also have an impact on your risk of type 2 diabetes. In the Nurses' Health Study, a 2% increase in trans fat consumption was associated with a 39% increased risk of type 2 diabetes (8). A 5% increase in polyunsaturated fat was associated with a

37% decreased risk of type 2 diabetes. Total fat, monounsaturated fat and saturated fat were not associated with risk of type 2 diabetes in this investigation.

Cancer

There is not a lot of strong evidence that dietary fat impacts risk of cancer in either direction. It is worth noting that in the younger Nurses' Health II cohort, women with the highest animal fat intake had a 33% increased risk of breast cancer (9). In this investigation, both red meat and high fat dairy were associated with an increased risk of breast cancer. Vegetable fat was not associated with risk of breast cancer.

Omega-3 Fatty Acids

Omega-3 fatty acids are a very special type of polyunsaturated fatty acid that has been shown to have a powerfully beneficial impact on our health. They are found in fish, canola oil, soybean oil, and walnuts. In the research literature, a high consumption of omega-3 fatty acids has been associated with significantly lower risk of heart disease (10) and stroke (11). In an analysis of The Cardiovascular Health Study, subjects consuming the most omega-3 fatty acids had a 27% lower risk of all-cause mortality when compared to those who consumed the least (12). Even more impressive is that the high omega-3 consumers lived an average of 2.2 years longer after age 65 than those with the lowest consumption of omega 3 fatty acids. It is a really good idea to include sources of omega-3 fatty acids in your diet regularly.

Nuts

Nuts are a really good source of healthy fat and have been associated in the research literature with a number of positive health outcomes. In the Nurses' Health Study, women who consumed more than five ounces of nuts per week had a 35% lower risk of heart disease when compared to women who consumed less than one ounce of nuts per week (13).

A similar result was found with type 2 diabetes. Women in the Nurses' Health Study who consumed five or more ounces of nuts per week had a 27% lower risk of type 2 diabetes compared to women who consumed less than one ounce of nuts per week (14). In addition to their healthy fat profiles, nuts are a good source of fiber, magnesium, vitamins, minerals, antioxidants and protein. I advise my clients to include nuts on their menu daily.

I hope it is becoming obvious that all fats are not created equal. Some, like trans fat and saturated fat, have been found to be harmful to our health. Others, like monounsaturated and polyunsaturated fats, can be beneficial to our health and there is no reason to avoid them. It makes sense that we would want to limit our intake of saturated and trans fat and increase our intake of the more healthful mono and polyunsaturated fats. Fat also has another great feature. It helps to stabilize your blood sugar by slowing down the rate of stomach emptying. With the addition of fat, carbohydrates you consume will have a much easier impact on your blood sugar. Remember, just as with protein, you want to be sure to include one source of fat at each and every meal. So here are the best choices and choices to avoid for our all too misunderstood friend dietary fat.

Good Sources Of Fat
Vegetable Oil: Olive oil, canola oil, corn oil, flaxseed oil, sunflower oil, safflower oil, peanut oil, and soybean

oil are all good choices here. I especially recommend olive oil because it is high in monounsaturated fat and canola oil because it is high in alpha-linoleic acid, a vegetable form of omega-3 fatty acid.

Nuts: Peanuts, almonds, walnuts, cashews, hazel nuts, pistachios, macadamia nuts and any other nut is a great choice for your source of healthy fat.

Nuts Butters: Peanut butter, almond butter, cashew butter and any other nut butter is a great choice for your fat as well.

Seeds: Pumpkin seeds and sunflower seeds are a less commonly eaten, but are good source of dietary fat.

Mayonnaise

Butter Substitutes: *Olivio, Smart Balance* and *Earth Balance* are butters made from vegetable oils. They taste great and are a good source of healthy fat.

Sources Of Fat To Strictly Limit
Full Fat Dairy: Cream, whole milk, whole cheese, full-fat yogurt and whole cottage cheese are high in saturated fat.

Butter: Is high in saturated fat and should be strictly limited.

Certain Vegetable Oils: Palm oil and coconut oil are high in saturated fat and should be limited.

Trans Fat: Thankfully, trans fat is working its way out of our food supply. You can still find it in a few products. It can be identified on food labels. Avoid this type of fat at all costs.

<u>ACTION STEPS FOR THIS CHAPTER</u>

1. Don't be afraid of dietary fat. When chosen wisely, it can improve your health and facilitate weight loss.
2. Stay away from the unhealthy trans and saturated fats.
3. Choose healthy mono- and polyunsaturated fats at each meal.

Chapter 5

Carbohydrate: The Most Important Macronutrient

I'll do my very best to make this chapter brief because I could write an entire book on how carbohydrates impact our weight and our health in general. If your goal is lasting weight loss, the type of carbohydrate that you put into your body is of the utmost importance. Pay very close attention to this chapter!

Let's start from the very top. So, what exactly is a carbohydrate? Carbohydrates are composed of carbon, hydrogen and oxygen in the ratio of 1 to 2 to 1. Simpler forms of carbohydrates are also known as sugars, while more complex forms of carbohydrate are called starches. The major function of carbohydrate is to provide energy for the body and to help prevent the breakdown of protein.

The type of carbohydrate that human beings consume has changed quite a bit over the years. While we were still evolving, the majority of carbohydrates we ate were fruits and vegetables in their whole form, beans, other legumes and grains that were highly unrefined. As humans became more civilized, this all changed and not for the better.

Back before refrigeration and food preservatives, the transport and storage of food was a huge problem. Whole grains contain a small amount of fat that shortens the amount of time it takes for the grain to spoil. By refining the grain, this fat is removed. Therefore, early attempts to refine grains were initiated by the noblest of intentions; to keep food edible longer so fewer people would starve.

Thankfully, for most of this country, starvation isn't a huge issue. If anything, there is too much food available. The American diet is currently about 50% carbo-hydrates, 80% of which is refined carbs such as sugars, refined starch and potatoes (1). Therefore, for the typical American, 40% of all calories consumed are refined carbohydrates and this is a very big problem.

Biochemistry 101

In the *Introduction To Diet Plan* chapter, we introduced the concept of glycemic index and how rapidly absorbed carbohydrates can have a negative impact on appetite, subsequent energy intake and consequently, your body weight. It is time to focus on this concept in a bit more detail.

Let's start with a very brief lesson on what happens to your blood sugar when you eat a carbohydrate. Once you consume a carbohydrate, your blood sugar levels begin to rise. Our body works within a relatively narrow frame of blood sugar. You've got a problem if it goes too high, and you've got a problem if it goes too low. For this reason, your body releases insulin to lower your blood sugar. The amount of insulin released depends on the type and amount of carbohydrate consumed. Some carbohydrates cause the release of large amounts of insulin, while others cause a smaller amount of insulin to be released.

When the right type of carbohydrate is consumed, insulin does its job well and lowers blood glucose to normal levels. However, when you eat the wrong type of carbohydrate, blood sugar spikes to unnaturally high levels. In response to these very high glucose levels, the body releases a similarly unnaturally high insulin level to bring it back down. In most of us, this large dose of insulin does its job too well and causes a reactive hypoglycemia. When this happens, your blood sugar actually drops below fasting levels.

To deal with this situation, your body releases the counter-regulatory hormones glucagon, epinephrine, cortisol and growth hormone in an effort to bring back up your blood sugar (2). These swings in blood glucose and hormone levels can have a strong impact on satiety, hunger, subsequent energy intake and consequently, your body weight. These unnatural swings can also impact your level of energy, your mood, your immune system and your risk of developing some of today's most deadly chronic diseases.

In summary, all carbohydrates are not created equal! Some will raise your blood sugar really high, really fast, causing the release of large amounts of insulin. Other carbohydrates have a more slow and gradual effect on your blood sugar and do not necessitate a large release of insulin. Enter the glycemic index, which we introduced earlier in *Chapter 2*.

The glycemic index was proposed by Dr. David Jenkins at the University of Toronto in 1981 as a way of classifying carbohydrates (3). Very simply, it gives a score as to how quickly and how severely a carbohydrate will raise your blood sugar. It all starts by feeding a group of subjects 50 grams of glucose (which is pure sugar) and measuring their blood sugar response. This is the baseline or reference measure. Next, the researchers feed the same people 50 grams of another type of carbohydrate, say a baked potato, and measure their blood sugar response once again.

The glycemic index number is the blood sugar response of that particular carbohydrate relative to the pure glucose reading. For example, the glycemic index of a white baked potato is 78. What that really means is when you eat equal amounts of a white baked potato and pure glucose, the potato results in 78% of the blood sugar response of the pure glucose. This test is repeated for all types of carbohydrate containing foods. A glycemic index of less than 50 is considered low. There is quite a bit of variability in how carbohydrate containing foods impact our blood sugar. The highest glycemic index foods are five times higher than the lowest glycemic index foods (2).

Take a look at this example. Notice how the higher glycemic carbohydrate causes dramatic increases in insulin and glucose levels compared to the lower glycemic carbohydrate.

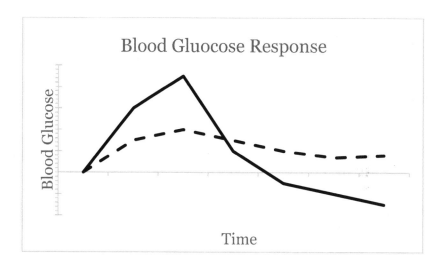

Blood Gluocose Response

Blood Glucose

Time

High Glycemic Carbohydrate
- - - - Low Glycemic Carbohydrate

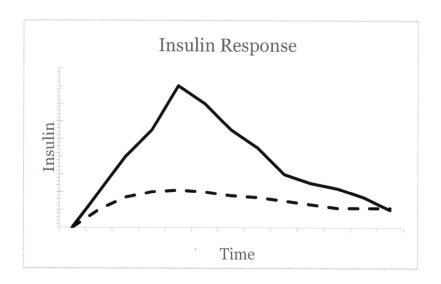

Insulin Response

Insulin

Time

We can use the glycemic index and a related concept called the glycemic load to help us pick our carbohydrates. The glycemic load was proposed by some of my colleagues at Harvard University and takes the concept of glycemic index one step further. The glycemic load is the glycemic index multiplied by the amount of carbohydrate supplied in a typical serving of the food. Therefore, the glycemic load takes into account both the quality and quantity of carbohydrate. In general, a food with a glycemic load of 10 or less is considered low glycemic load. A food with a glycemic load between 11 and 19 is considered moderate glycemic load. A food with a glycemic load of 20 or higher is considered a high glycemic load food.

Why is this extra step so important? Well, for starters, the glycemic load gives you a more practical look at how a carbohydrate will affect your blood sugar. Most of the foods that have a high glycemic index also have a high glycemic load. For example, white rice has a glycemic index of 91, which is considered very high and a glycemic load of 24.8, also considered very high. White bread has a glycemic index of 70 and a glycemic load of 21, both considered high. On the other end of the spectrum, lentil beans have a low glycemic index of 29 and also a low glycemic load of 5.7 and apples similarly have both a low glycemic index (36) and a low glycemic load (8.1).

However, there are some interesting exceptions. Carrots have a high glycemic index at 71 but the glycemic load of carrots is small at 3.8. This is because carrots have a lot of fiber and water and supply only a small amount of carbohydrate per serving. Hence the lower glycemic load. Remember, glycemic load is the product of both the glycemic index and the amount of carbohydrate.

So, you can see that some foods with a high glycemic index really won't hurt your blood sugar because only small amounts of carbohydrate are delivered. On the other hand, some foods with more moderate glycemic indices, like pasta, will really hurt your blood sugar because of the large amount of carbohydrates delivered in a serving. To aid in the weight loss process, you want to focus on foods with a low glycemic load.

It should not come as a huge surprise that the overwhelming majority of foods with a high glycemic load are man-made, refined carbohydrates. The big offenders are bread, pasta, white rice and sugar. Most fruits and vegetables have a much lower glycemic load and will have a milder effect on your blood sugar. This makes sense because fruits, vegetables and legumes are the carbohydrates that were put on the Earth for us to consume. These foods are what we evolved with and it is not surprising that our bodies function best when consuming them.

The glycemic load and the glycemic index are amazing tools to help us pick our carbohydrates. However, you want to use them more as a guide than as an absolute rule. Carbohydrate quality is just one of several things to consider when picking foods.

A good example of this is full fat premium ice cream. It has a low glycemic index of 37 and a low glycemic load of 4 (for a 50 gram serving). However, it contains a lot of saturated fat and sugar and should be avoided for these reasons.

Similarly, whole grains like brown rice, oatmeal and quinoa can have moderately high glycemic loads. They are also a great source of fiber, antioxidants, phyto-estrogens and minerals like magnesium, selenium, copper and manganese. Whole grains have been associated with a reduced risk of heart disease, diabetes and certain cancers (4). It would be a mistake to eliminate whole grains from your diet because they are not super low on the glycemic load scale. Having said this and despite a few notable exceptions, glycemic load is a very important tool to help you pick healthy carbs.

When choosing what carbohydrates to eat, we want to focus on lower glycemic load carbohydrates like fruits, vegetables, legumes and whole grains such as brown rice, quinoa and oatmeal. There are just a few small exceptions. For fruits, go a little easier on bananas and grapes. They have less fiber than other fruits and are, therefore, higher glycemic. Certainly, don't eliminate them from your diet, just don't make them a daily choice. For vegetables, the only notable exception is white potatoes. They are really high glycemic and should be consumed with moderation. Always keep in mind Rule #1: You want to combine your low glycemic load carbohydrate with a healthy source of fat and protein at each and every meal.

Determinants Of A Food's Glycemic Index

Increases GI	Decreases GI
Processing/Refining food	Addition of fat
Longer cooking times	Addition of protein
	Addition of fiber

As a side note, consuming a diet with a high glycemic load has been shown to increase your risk of chronic disease. Let's take a quick look at some of this research.

Health Effects Of Carbohydrates

Heart Disease

I personally published a paper in 2006 that examined the association between glycemic load and risk of coronary heart disease in women from The Nurses' Health Study. We followed 82,802 women for 20 years, during which time we documented 1,994 new cases of coronary heart disease (5). Women with the highest dietary glycemic load had a 90% increased risk of heart disease compared to women with the lowest glycemic load. We believed that the increased risk was due to the negative impact on HDL cholesterol, triglycerides and insulin sensitivity that is often seen with high glycemic load diets.

The association between glycemic load and cardio-vascular disease was examined in 15,714 Dutch women in the European Prospective Investigation Into Cancer And Nutrition (EPIC) cohort. After 9 years, women with the highest dietary glycemic load had a 47% increased risk of cardiovascular disease when compared to women with the lowest dietary glycemic load (6). The researchers attributed the increased risk to the detrimental effects of high glycemic load diets on insulin sensitivity and blood lipid profiles.

If you need more evidence, a meta-analysis that included 10 studies and over 240,000 subjects showed that those with the highest GL had a 27% higher risk of heart disease compared to those with the lowest GL (7). The results were particularly pronounced for women in this study.

Diabetes

I published a study that looked at the association between glycemic load and risk of type 2 diabetes in

85,059 women from the Nurses' Health Study (8). Over 20 years of follow-up, there were 4,670 new cases of type 2 diabetes. Women with the highest dietary glycemic load had 2½ times the risk of type 2 diabetes when compared to women with the lowest dietary glycemic load. We hypothesized that the lower glycemic load diet offered protection due to its decreased glucose and insulin response, lowered glycated hemoglobin, and improved insulin sensitivity.

In an updated analysis of over 200,000 subjects that included three Harvard cohorts (The Nurses' Health Study, The Health Professionals Follow-up Study and The Nurses' Health Study II) over 18 years of follow-up, both the glycemic index and the glycemic load were significantly associated with an increased risk of diabetes (9). Subjects with a combination of a high glycemic load diet and low cereal fiber had a 47% increased risk of diabetes. This study also included a meta-analysis of 14 studies, showing that subjects in the highest category of glycemic load had a significantly higher risk of type 2 diabetes.

Stroke

The association between dietary glycemic load and risk of stroke was examined in the Nurses' Health Study in 2005 (10). Over 78,000 women were followed for 18 years, during which time there were 1,020 new cases of stroke. Among women with a BMI of 25 or higher, glycemic load was associated with a 61% increased risk of stroke. This association was not seen in women of normal weight. The combination of a high glycemic load diet and overweight seemed to be the most harmful. The researchers theorized that the increased risk seen with the higher glycemic load diet was due to decreases in

HDL cholesterol, increases in blood pressure, C-reactive protein and insulin resistance. All of these factors tend to increase risk of stroke.

Cancer

There is not a lot of research on glycemic load and cancer, but one study is worth mentioning. The association between glycemic load and colon cancer was assessed in the Women's Health Study cohort (11). Over 38,000 women were followed for eight years. Women with the highest dietary glycemic load had almost 3 times the risk of developing colon cancer when compared to women with the lowest glycemic load. The researchers believed that the higher rate of cancer was due to higher insulin derived growth factor levels in women with the high glycemic load diets. This hormone is thought to stimulate mitosis and cell proliferation.

The considerable health benefits of consuming a low glycemic load diet are reason enough to change your source of carbohydrates. Now let's take a look at how choosing the right carbs makes it so much easier to lose weight.

Impact Of Carbohydrates On Body Weight

There has been a considerable amount of research on how carbohydrate quality can impact weight. In one fascinating study, 12 obese teenage boys were given test meals on 3 separate occasions. The meals were identical in total calories but differed in a very important way. One was high glycemic index, one was low glycemic index and one was medium glycemic index (12). For 5 hours after the test meal, subjects had access to an all you can eat lunch buffet. Voluntary energy intake after eating the high glycemic index meal was 53% greater than after eating the medium glycemic index test meal and was 81% greater than after eating the low glycemic index test meal. Not surprisingly, ratings of hunger after the test meal were higher after the high GI meal compared to the low GI meal at all time points.

Earlier, in Chapter 2, I referenced a study that is worth repeating. In an investigation of more than 120,000 men and women from Harvard School of Public Health cohorts, researchers found that many of the foods associated with long-term weight gain had a high glycemic index (13). This list included refined grains, sweets and desserts, sugar-sweetened beverages, potatoes, French fries and potato chips. It is no surprise that many of the foods that were significantly associated with weight loss were low glycemic, including fruits, vegetables and whole grains.

There is also evidence that foods with a high glycemic index are addictive. In a fascinating study published in *The American Journal of Clinical Nutrition*, 12 overweight men consumed a high glycemic index and a low glycemic index meal on two separate occasions (14). The meals were identical with regards to calories, macronutrients and palatability. After 4 hours, hunger was significantly greater after the high glycemic index meal.

Furthermore, after undergoing an MRI of the brain, the high glycemic index meal elicited significantly greater brain activity in the right nucleus accumbens, a part of the brain associated with reward and craving. This part of the brain is also involved in substance abuse and dependence, which led the researchers to conclude that high glycemic index carbs may actually be addictive.

One would assume that with less hunger, subsequent energy intake and food-addictive behavior, we should see increased weight loss with a low glycemic load approach. Several studies have demonstrated this. In 28 obese young adults with high fasting insulin levels, subjects randomized to a low glycemic load diet lost over 10 lbs. more than those randomized to a low-fat diet after 18 months (15).

Similarly, in a randomized crossover trial, 16 subjects lost 6½ more pounds after 12 weeks on a low glycemic diet compared to a high glycemic diet (16). In a randomized crossover trial that included 11 healthy young men, subjects had a significantly lower fat mass after 5 weeks on a low glycemic index diet compared to 5 weeks on a high glycemic index diet (17).

Finally, a retrospective cohort study of 107 obese children compared the weight loss impact of a low glycemic index diet and a low-fat diet (18). After 4 months, the children on the low glycemic index diet lost 4.5 lbs., while the children on the low-fat diet actually gained 2.9 pounds. Body mass index was also reduced by 1.47 units in the low glycemic index group compared to the low-fat group. Both of these differences were statistically significant.

Now that we have learned a bit about the science and research concerning carbohydrates, here are the best choices and the carbs to avoid.

Good Sources Of Carbohydrate
Fruits And Vegetables: The majority of fruits and vegetables are easy on your blood sugar and are an excellent source of dietary carbohydrate. There are just a few notable exceptions:

-Bananas and grapes have a higher glycemic load than most other fruits, so go easy on them.

-It is also important to strictly limit white potatoes, which really spike blood sugar.

-All other fruits and vegetables are permitted.

-Strictly limit fruit and vegetable juices as well as dried fruits, such as raisins and dried cranberries. These can also really spike the blood sugar.

Whole Grains: These are a health promoting and delicious carb choice. Old fashioned oatmeal, steel cut oats and Irish oatmeal are a great choice for breakfast. Just be sure to avoid instant or quick cooking oats, which are a bit tougher on your blood sugar due to the additional processing they undergo. Brown rice, quinoa and corn are other good sources of whole grains.

Beans And Other Legumes: Black beans, pink beans, chick peas, hummus, lentils and any other bean are a great choice of low glycemic carbohydrate.

Sources Of Carbohydrate To Strictly Limit
Bread: Limit white bread, wheat bread, wraps, pita bread, flour tortillas, bagels, crackers and pretzels. While we are talking about snack foods, limit popcorn as well.

Pasta

White Rice: Also be sure to limit white rice products like rice cakes and rice crackers.

White Potatoes: And potato products like potato chips.

Sugar: Strictly limit all sources of added sugar, including cakes, cookies, candy, pies, donuts, soda, jelly, jams, sweetened yogurts and high sugar condiments like ketchup, barbecue sauce and steak sauce.

Right about now you may be saying "I'll never be able to give up bread and sugar! I crave them way too much!" Many people feel this way at the beginning of the program and I will admit that at first it is a challenge to give up these foods. However, it is important to know that when your blood sugar becomes more stable, usually in just a few weeks, these cravings will go away entirely. I haven't had sugar in over 20 years now and believe me when I tell you I don't even think twice about it anymore; and I had the biggest sweet tooth on Long Island when I was a kid.

In my personal experience and that of my clients, cravings for these refined carbohydrate foods are not psychological but physiological. When you are in "bad blood sugar" you often crave quick release carbohydrates to counter the dip in blood glucose caused by higher levels of insulin. It truly is a vicious cycle. When you are in a state of "good blood sugar" these cravings disappear. It is not a question of mental strength or mental weakness. Stabilize your blood sugar and the cravings go away.

Americans consume a lot of sugar. We average 20 teaspoons a day, which is over 300 calories. Many people are actually addicted to sugar and other refined carbohydrates and go through a withdrawal period when giving them up. We have seen in this chapter research evidence of just how addictive sugar and refined carbs can be. In the first few weeks of eliminating sugar and refined carbohydrates from your diet, you may notice that you are a little more tired and irritable and may even get a headache or two. You'll also have some serious cravings for the foods you are limiting. These symptoms are not serious and will go away on their own after 2 to 3 weeks on the program.

After a few weeks of eating this way, you can once again listen to your hunger to tell you what your body needs. You will no longer get hungry in order to fix your blood sugar. Although it is a bit rough at first, one of the biggest surprises for my clients is that they no longer crave bread, pasta, white rice and sugar after just a few weeks. You'll get there too! You just need to tough it out for the first 14 days or so.

Hidden Sugars

Sugar is everywhere! To avoid it, you must become a big time label reader. For example, ketchup, barbeque sauce, steak sauce and low-fat salad dressings are loaded with sugar and need to be avoided. Thankfully, today's food labels are much easier to read than in years past. In 2016, the FDA passed a law requiring food manufacturers to list added sugars in a separate category on food labels. Previously, there was a listing for total sugars that included both natural and added sugars. This was quite confusing for some foods, particularly dairy foods.

Dairy foods naturally contain a low glycemic sugar called lactose that does not cause any problems with blood glucose levels. Under the old food labels, a glass of milk would have 12 grams of sugar listed on the food label under "Sugars". This wasn't added sugar but a naturally occurring sugar. Generally, natural sugars are not a problem, added sugars are what you are looking to limit. The addition of "Added Sugars" to food labels is a huge step forward.

Below is an example of a typical food label. Look under the "Total Carbohydrate" category and you'll see a listing for "Total Sugars" and under that, one for "Added Sugars". The one to pay attention to is "Added Sugars". You want this number to be as close to 0 as possible. Divide this number by 4 and that is the number of teaspoons of sugar found in a serving of that food. In our example there are 10 grams of added sugar per serving (2½ teaspoons). Stay away from this food for sure!

Nutrition Facts

8 servings per container

Serving size   2/3 cup (55g)

Amount per serving

Calories   230

	% Daily Value*
Total Fat 8g	**10%**
Saturated Fat 1g	**5%**
Trans Fat 0g	
Cholesterol 0mg	**0%**
Sodium 160mg	**7%**
Total Carbohydrate 37g	**13%**
Dietary Fiber 4g	**14%**
Total Sugars 12g	
Includes 10g Added Sugars	**20%**
Protein 3g	
Vitamin D 2mcg	10%
Calcium 260mg	20%
Iron 8mg	45%
Potassium 235mg	6%

* The % Daily Value (DV) tells you how much a nutrient in a serving of food contributes to a daily diet. 2,000 calories a day is used for general nutrition advice.

Food manufacturers use lots of different names for sugars. Following is a list of ingredients that basically can be translated to SUGAR. This is important when reading food labels, rarely will you see the word "sugar" listed as an ingredient.

> Sucrose
> Molasses
> Concentrated Fruit Juice
> Corn Syrup
> Corn Sweetener
> Brown Sugar
> Raw Sugar
> Cane Syrup
> High Fructose Corn Syrup
> Dextrose
> Fructose
> Levulose
> Maple Sugar
> Turbinado
> Honey
> Dextrin
> Glucose
> Galactose
> Maltose
> Beet Sugar
> Cane Sugar

So, there you have it. Carbohydrate quality and quantity are crucial to understand if you are attempting to lose weight. In my opinion, the combination of high glycemic load carbohydrates and low-fat diets have much to do with the explosion of obesity in recent years.

Decreases in physical activity also play a huge role. But we'll get to that a little bit later!

ACTION STEPS FOR THIS CHAPTER

1. As always, combine a source of fat, protein and carbohydrate at every meal.
2. Focus on low glycemic load carbohydrates from the "Good Sources of Carbohydrates" list.
3. Become a label reader.
4. Beware of hidden sources of sugars in the foods you eat.
5. Become familiar with all of the words manufacturers use for sugar.

Chapter 6

Putting It All Together

You now should have a very good idea of what type of foods to eat and what type of foods to limit in order to lose weight and improve your health. It is time to put it all together. I have said it before, and I'll say it again; The most important thing to remember is the following:

Every time you eat, make sure to pick one healthy carb, one healthy fat and one healthy protein.

If you do this regularly, you'll accomplish several goals:

1. You will be sure to get enough healthy fat in your diet.
2. You will be sure to get adequate protein in your diet.
3. Most importantly, you will have a stable blood sugar. As we have learned, a stable blood sugar will decrease your hunger, reduce cravings for refined carbs and result in a much lower energy intake. Blood sugar stability will also even out swings in insulin levels, which promote a fat burning environment, rather than a fat storing environment.

This is really easy to accomplish. Just keep in mind all of the healthy proteins, fats and carbs that we learned in the last few chapters. When planning a meal, pick one food from each list. Do your best to vary them on a day to day basis but definitely let your tastes guide you. Let's say this is day one of your new life. Logically, breakfast is a great place to start since it is the first meal of the day. Pick a breakfast protein from the list of acceptable protein foods, say nonfat plain yogurt. Now move over to the fat category and select whatever you want, some peanuts, for example. Lastly look at the carbohydrate group and pick a food, some cantaloupe will do nicely. We will worry about portions in just a minute. For now, understand the choice of a food from each category as being a critical part of the dietary regimen.

Breakfast
Protein--Plain nonfat yogurt
Fat--Peanuts
Carbohydrate--Cantaloupe

Lunch
Protein--Grilled chicken
Fat--Olive oil
Carbohydrate--Salad vegetables

Dinner
Protein--Salmon
Fat--Canola oil
Carbohydrate--Brown rice and broccoli

Now let's move to lunch. An ideal lunch would be the following: a big salad with lots of vegetables (carbo-hydrate), some grilled chicken on top (protein) and some olive oil and vinegar dressing (fat). Get the idea? One from each category, any one you want. How about dinner? Let's start with a nice piece of salmon (protein), some brown rice and broccoli sautéed in canola oil (carbohydrate and fat).

Pretty easy, right? It will take a little getting used to but once you get going, you'll find it is a flexible way to eat filled with a variety of delicious and health promoting foods. Following are a few more sample days on the plan.

Day 1: Monday

Breakfast
Plain non-fat yogurt
Peanuts
Sliced cantaloupe

*The yogurt provides the protein. The nuts provide the fat.
The cantaloupe provides the carbohydrate.*

Lunch
Chicken vegetable soup with brown rice
Apple

*The chicken provides the protein. The oil in the soup
provides the fat. The vegetables, brown rice and apple
provide the carbohydrate.*

Dinner
Grilled salmon
Brown rice
Broccoli sautéed in canola oil.

*The salmon provides the protein. The canola oil provides
the fat. The brown rice and broccoli provide the carbohydrate.*

Day 2: Tuesday

Breakfast
Oatmeal made with milk and topped with walnuts
Blueberries

*The milk provides the protein. The walnuts provide the fat. The oatmeal and blueberries provide the carbohydrate.

Lunch
Tuna pouch
Sweet potato
Almonds
Grapefruit

*The tuna pouch provides the protein. The almonds provide the fat. The sweet potato and grapefruit provide the carbohydrate.

Dinner
Chicken enchiladas (chicken, olive oil, black beans, corn and onion in a soft corn tortilla topped with salsa).

*The chicken provides the protein. The olive oil provides the fat. The vegetables and whole grain corn tortillas provide the carbohydrate.

Day 3: Wednesday

Breakfast
Scrambled eggs
Raspberries

The eggs provide the protein and fat. The raspberries provide the carbohydrate.

Lunch
Brown rice sushi with avocado
Pineapple slices

The fish provides the protein. The avocado provides the fat. The brown rice and the pineapple provide the carbohydrate.

Dinner
Splurge ☺

Twice a week, you are allowed to have a splurge meal and go off the diet a bit. We'll learn more about this in Chapter 10.

Day 4: Thursday

Breakfast
Oatmeal (made with water and not milk)
Turkey bacon (nitrate free and low sodium)
Pistachio nuts
Strawberries

The turkey provides the protein. The pistachio nuts provide the fat. The oatmeal and strawberries provide the carbohydrate.

Lunch
Grilled shrimp garden salad
Olive oil and vinegar dressing
Sliced mango

The shrimp provide the protein. The olive oil provides the fat. The salad vegetables and mango provide the carbohydrate.

Dinner
Chicken fajitas with a side of black beans
Soft corn tortillas

The chicken provides the protein. The canola oil (to sauté the vegetables) provides the fat. The fajita vegetables (onion, pepper, tomato), black beans and corn tortillas provide the carbohydrate.

Day 5: Friday

Breakfast
Low fat cottage cheese
Grapefruit
Cashews

The cottage cheese provides the protein. The cashews provide the fat. The grapefruit provides the carbohydrate.

Lunch
Lentil soup
Orange

The lentils provide the protein. The vegetable oil in the soup provides the fat. The lentils, vegetables, and orange provide the carbohydrate.

Dinner
Lean ground beef burger with tomato and onion
(Without the roll)
Black bean and corn salad
Sweet potato fries

The burger provides the protein. The oil in the black bean and corn salad provides the fat. The onions, tomato, beans, corn, and sweet potato provide the carbohydrate.

Day 6: Saturday

Breakfast
Oatmeal made with low fat milk
Almond butter
Watermelon

The milk provides the protein. The almond butter provides the fat. The oatmeal and the watermelon provide the carbohydrate.

Lunch
Grilled chicken garden salad
Italian dressing
Orange

The chicken provides the protein. The salad vegetables and orange provide the carbohydrate. The olive oil in the salad dressing provides the fat.

Dinner
Splurge ☺

Day 7: Sunday

Breakfast
Vegetable omelet
Sliced kiwi

The eggs provide the protein and fat. The vegetables and kiwi provide the carbohydrate.

Lunch
Garden salad with sliced turkey breast
Italian dressing
Pear

The turkey provides the protein. The oil in the dressing provides the fat. The salad vegetables and pear provide the carbohydrate.

Dinner
Chicken stir fry
Brown rice

The chicken provides the protein. The olive oil used in the stir fry provides the fat. The brown rice and vegetables provide the carbohydrate.

Day 8: Monday

Breakfast
Hardboiled eggs
Strawberries

The eggs provide the protein and fat. The strawberries provide the carbohydrate.

Lunch
Grilled chicken garden salad
Olive oil and vinegar
Sliced watermelon

The chicken provides the protein. The olive oil provides the fat. The salad vegetables and watermelon provide the carbohydrate.

Dinner
Shrimp Scampi
Quinoa
Steamed broccoli and red peppers

The shrimp provides the protein. The olive oil in the Scampi sauce provides the fat. The quinoa and vegetables provide the carbohydrate.

Day 9: Tuesday

Breakfast
Low fat mozzarella cheese sticks
Pistachio nuts
Apple

The mozzarella cheese provides the protein. The pistachios provide the fat. The apple provides the carbohydrate.

Lunch
Romaine lettuce and tomato turkey roll-ups
Almonds
Pear

The turkey provides the protein. The almonds provide the fat. The lettuce, tomato, and pear provide the carbohydrate.

Dinner
Healthy chicken tacos (hard corn tortilla shells with chicken, lettuce, tomatoes, onion, black beans, corn and olive oil to sauté the vegetables)

The chicken provides the protein. The lettuce, tomatoes, onion, black beans and corn taco shell provide the carbohydrate. The olive oil and corn taco shell provide the fat.

Day 10: Wednesday

Breakfast
Breakfast tacos (scrambled eggs, low fat cheese, turkey sausage and salsa wrapped in a soft corn tortilla)
Cantaloupe

The eggs, low-fat cheese, and turkey sausage provide the protein. The eggs provide the fat. The soft corn tortillas and salsa provide the carbohydrate.

Lunch
Tuna salad
Apple

The tuna provides the protein. The apple provides the carbohydrate. The mayonnaise provides the fat.

Dinner
Splurge ☺

Day 11: Thursday

Breakfast
Vanilla almond butter oatmeal (oatmeal made with low fat milk, vanilla extract, almond butter and topped with cinnamon)
Blueberries

The low-fat milk provides the protein. The almond butter provides the fat. The oatmeal and blueberries provide the carbohydrate.

Lunch
Garden salad with sliced turkey breast
Olive oil and vinegar dressing
Orange

The turkey provides the protein. The olive oil provides the fat. The salad vegetables and orange provide the carbohydrate.

Dinner
Turkey burger (without the roll)
Black bean and corn salad
Steamed vegetables

The turkey burger provides the protein. The beans, corn, and vegetables provide the carbohydrate. The olive oil in the black bean and corn salad provides the fat.

Day 12: Friday

Breakfast
Plain non-fat yogurt
Walnuts
Sliced pineapple

The yogurt provides the protein. The walnuts provide the fat. The pineapple provides the carbohydrate.

Lunch
Tuna salad made with white beans, onions, olive oil and vinegar
Sliced kiwi

The beans and tuna provide the protein. The beans, onion, and kiwi provide the carbohydrate. The olive oil provides the fat.

Dinner
Crab cakes with mango salsa
Quinoa
Steamed vegetables

The crab provides the protein. The quinoa, mango, and vegetables provide the carbohydrate. The oil in the mango salsa and the egg provide the fat.

Day 13: Saturday

Breakfast
Oatmeal made with low-fat milk and peanut butter
Grapefruit half

The low-fat milk provides the protein. The peanut butter provides the fat. The oatmeal and grapefruit provide the carbohydrate.

Lunch
Turkey chili
Peach

The turkey and beans provide the protein. The beans, vegetables, and peach provide the carbohydrate. The olive oil in the chili provides the fat.

Dinner
Splurge ☺

Day 14: Sunday

Breakfast
Poached eggs with Canadian bacon
Raspberries

The eggs and Canadian bacon provide the protein. The eggs provide the fat. The raspberries provide the carbohydrate.

Lunch
Chicken salad with walnuts and apple over salad greens

The chicken provides the protein. The mayonnaise and walnuts provide the fat. The apple and lettuce provide the carbohydrate.

Dinner
Grilled filet mignon
Brown rice
Broccoli and cauliflower sautéed in olive oil

The filet provides the protein. The olive oil provides the fat. The brown rice, broccoli and cauliflower provide the carbohydrate.

Notes On Meal Planning

While working with clients over the last 20 years, I've learned quite a bit about different eating styles. I've had clients that take the time to prepare gourmet recipes. Others have needed very quick meal prep times. Some people are on a tight budget and are looking to limit their food expenditures. There are people that need to eat meals in their car, on a plane, or in two minutes between meetings. Despite these lifestyle differences, all of these people shared one common goal—to get control of their eating, lose weight and keep it off for good.

In reality, most of my clients are all of these people at one time or another. Different career, family, and travel situations can change our eating patterns from week to week and even day to day. Therefore, my goal when creating this meal plan was to create solutions for all of these circumstances.

It is my sincere hope that you will find a meal option for whatever life throws your way. I've included meals that can be eaten on the go, meals with very quick prep times, meals on a budget, and also a few meals for those occasions when you have the time and desire to make your food very special.

How To Use This Meal Plan

There are several ways to use this meal plan. If you want to follow it exactly, day by day and meal by meal, your diet will be just about perfect! However, you can also use the meal plan more as a guide, picking meals here and there that suit your tastes and current lifestyle needs.

If you decide to follow the meal plan exactly, all of the thinking has been done for you. If you decide to use the meal plan as more of a guide, keep in mind that the plan has been built around a number of key guidelines that you'll want to follow. These guidelines are in place to help reduce your risk of chronic disease, as well as facilitate permanent weight loss.

1) Aim for 1-2 servings of whole grains each day. Whole grains have been shown to have a multitude of health benefits, including reducing the risk of heart disease, stroke, type 2 diabetes, and certain cancers. Examples of whole grains are brown rice, oatmeal, quinoa, and whole grain corn tortillas.

2) Limit egg yolks to 6 per week. Eggs are a great food. The yolks, although often criticized, actually provide a lot of vitamins, minerals, and other nutrients. They are very much like a multivitamin pill. Consuming up to 6 or 7 yolks per week has been shown to be safe in the research literature. However, due to their high cholesterol content, you don't want to go overboard with egg yolks, so don't go higher than that. If you have diabetes, it is a good idea to strictly limit egg yolk consumption. Some research has shown an increased risk of heart disease in diabetics who consumed a lot of egg yolks.

3) Limit dairy to around 5 servings per week. Dairy has always been a tough one for me as a nutritionist. I'm not a big fan of dairy products. From an evolutionary standpoint, we are the only animal to drink milk after six months, and the only species to drink another species' milk. The protein in milk was designed for a totally different digestive system than ours. Cows have four stomachs! I don't think milk is the most natural food for us. I've also found that many of my clients are lactose intolerant or have other, less obvious sensitivities to milk. In general, most of my clients will report a benefit when reducing their dairy consumption.

On the other hand, milk is one of the best sources of calcium in our diets. Calcium is important for lots of reasons, including ensuring strong bones. Therefore, I like to include some dairy in my clients' diets, but not too much. A good compromise is 4 to 5 servings per week.

4) *Limit red meat to 1 serving per week.* I don't think there is a need to completely eliminate red meat. Lean cuts, like filet mignon or 90% lean ground beef, are fine once a week, and provide a good source of iron that is highly absorbable. However, eating too much red meat has been associated with an increased risk of certain diseases, including heart disease and colon cancer. The relationship with colon cancer is likely due to carcinogenic heterocyclic amines that form during the cooking of red meat. So, if you are picking and choosing meals from the plan instead of following it to the letter, try not to include more than one red meat meal per week. Processed red meats like bacon, hot dogs, pepperoni, salami, and other fatty deli meats are particularly harmful. Be sure to strictly limit these foods.

5) *Shoot for seafood 3-4 times per week, but not much more than that.* Seafood is our best source of omega 3 fatty acids. These special polyunsaturated fats have been shown to have a beneficial impact on risk of heart disease, stroke, and even some cancers. However, good sources of marine omega 3's are often good sources of mercury. Mercury is a toxic metal that accumulates in

predatory fish and can cause neurological problems in adults, children, and developing fetuses. To keep mercury levels low, avoid the biggest sources: tilefish, swordfish, shark, albacore tuna, and king mackerel. Also, keep total seafood intake to 3-4 times per week. If you are pregnant, trying to become pregnant, or nursing, talk to your doctor about the amount of seafood you should include in your diet.

6) *Shoot for at least 5 servings of fruits and vegetables each day—more is better.* Fruits and vegetables are the healthiest things that you can eat. They are high in vitamins, minerals, fiber, antioxidants and other phytochemicals. People who eat a lot of fruits and vegetables have lower risks of heart disease, stroke, obesity, type 2 diabetes, hypertension, and other conditions. Try to have a piece of fruit with breakfast and lunch and vegetables everywhere that you can squeeze them in.

7) *Get a variety of fruits and vegetables.* You've probably noticed that on the meal plan, I have really tried to vary the fruit and vegetable selections. This was no accident. Each fruit and vegetable has its own unique combination of vitamins, minerals, phytochemicals, and antioxidants. To get the whole spectrum, you really want to eat as many varieties as you can. Having said this, let your tastes guide you. If a meal calls for a pear and you just can't stand them, it is OK to substitute another fruit. Just try to eat as many different fruits and vegetables as possible.

8) *Eat a serving of nuts just about every day.* Although often criticized for their high fat content, nuts are an extremely healthy food. They are a good source of poly-

and monounsaturated fat, protein, fiber, vitamins, and minerals. They are also low glycemic load and therefore very easy on the blood sugar. Nuts have been shown to reduce the risk of heart disease and type 2 diabetes in the research literature. Nut butters are also a great choice. You do need to watch the portions because they are very high in calories.

9) *Include legumes with your meals at least 4 times per week.* Legumes are a great source of protein and low glycemic carbohydrate. They are high in fiber and really good for you. Make sure you include some black beans, kidney beans, pink beans, lentil soup, hummus, or other legumes at least 4 times per week.

Portions

I never have my clients weigh their food or get too crazy about portion sizes, but a few guidelines are really important. Let's look at each of the macronutrients and talk a bit about portion sizes.

Protein

While at Harvard, a fair amount of my research was focused on low carbohydrate diets, like Atkins. On a low carb diet, protein is allowed in unlimited quantities and you are encouraged to eat as much as you want. In randomized trials studying people consuming a low carb diet, I found it interesting that protein intake never really exceeded 20-25% of calories. These people were allowed to eat as much protein as they wanted to and yet they really didn't go overboard. I have noticed the same thing with my clients.

The reason for this ends up being quite simple. Protein contains nitrogen, which is difficult for the human body to process and can be quite toxic at high levels. For this reason, the body tends to limit the protein that it will have to process. In other words, you won't overeat protein. So, the take home message here regarding protein portions is to eat protein until you are full. Your body won't let you go higher than 20-25% of calories, which is just where I want you to be.

Carbohydrates

The vast majority of carbohydrates on this plan are very low in calories. Fruits and vegetables contain a lot of fiber and water. For this reason, there really are no limits to the amounts of fruits, vegetables and other allowable carbs on this program. Eat until you are full. A bowl of broccoli will run you about 130 calories while the same size bowl of pasta can be 600 calories. Load up on a wide variety of fruits and vegetables without stressing too much about portions.

Fats

Fat is the only macronutrient that has strict portion guidelines. Having too little fat in your diet will cause you to have blood sugar issues. Having too much fat in your diet will cause you to have calorie issues. Follow these portions to avoid both scenarios. Please note that these portions are per meal, not per day.

For Women
1. If you are having oil, mayo or butter substitute, 1 tablespoon will do it.

2. If you are having nuts, 7 large nuts (cashews, macadamia nuts, walnuts, almonds) will do, 14 small nuts like peanuts or pistachio nuts will do.
3. If you are having nut butter, 1 tablespoon.
4. If you are having avocado as your fat source, ¼ if it's a large avocado and ½ if it's a small avocado.

For Men
1. If you are having oil, mayo or butter substitute, 1½ tablespoons will do it.
2. Nuts: 12 large and 24 small.
3. Nut butter: 1½ tablespoons.
4. Avocado: ½ if it's a large avocado and ¾ if it's a small avocado.

A Note Concerning Beans And Eggs

Most foods fit neatly into either the protein, fat or carbohydrate category. A few foods overlap and really fit into 2 groups. Eggs, eaten whole with the yolk, provide both protein and fat. Therefore, if you have eggs at a meal, they will satisfy both your protein and fat requirement and all you'll need is a carb. If you are only using the egg whites, then count them just as your protein. Beans and other legumes similarly are a good source of both protein and carbohydrate and should be counted as a source of both when planning meals.

Good Foods To Always Keep On Hand

As you can see, this program allows a lot of freedom to choose foods you enjoy, foods that taste great and have the benefits of not only helping you lose weight but increasing your energy and health in general. It is important to think about your meals well ahead of time and when you shop, make sure you have all the tools you need to construct your meal plan for the day. It's always a good idea to keep the following items well stocked in order to stay on track.

Proteins- sliced turkey breast, tuna, eggs, chicken, beans, low fat dairy such as plain non-fat yogurt, skim milk and low-fat cottage cheese.

Fats- olive oil, canola oil, peanut butter, nuts, seeds and a nice oil-based butter substitute like Olivio or Smart Balance.

Carbohydrates- a wide variety of fruits and vegetables, beans, old fashioned slow cooked oatmeal, brown rice and quinoa.

If you need a quick meal, grab a few slices of turkey breast, a handful of nuts and an apple and you're out the door. If you need a quick breakfast when running late for work, have a few spoonfuls of low-fat cottage cheese or plain non-fat yogurt, grab some sunflower seeds and a pear and you're on your way.

The key is to always keep on hand the raw materials you need to build your meals. We all run into trouble when we have nothing in the house and stop for something on the way to work. What you grab for convenience is almost never as good as what you'd have if you took a little time to plan your meals.

So, this concludes the all-important dietary component of the plan. Now it is time to focus our attention on the two exercise components of the program: cardiovascular training and resistance training.

ACTION STEPS FOR THIS CHAPTER

1. Combine a fat, a protein and a carbohydrate at each meal.
2. When it comes to protein and carbohydrate, don't worry much about portions. Eat until you are full. Once your blood sugar stabilizes, your hunger will reflect what your body needs.
3. Strictly follow the fat portions. Too little fat and you'll have blood sugar issues, too much fat and you'll have calorie issues.
4. Remember that eggs with the yolks will count as both your fat and your protein and beans count as both your protein and carbohydrate.
5. Keep your pantry stocked with all you will need to construct blood sugar stabilizing meals. Preparation is critical to success.

Chapter 7

Cardiovascular Exercise

After your diet, cardiovascular exercise is the 2nd most important factor that will determine your weight loss success. First of all, cardio burns calories. This will help to access the undesirable fat stores you are looking to reduce. Believe it or not, this isn't even the major benefit of cardiovascular exercise. For about 24 hours after a cardio session, you burn more calories than you would if you had not exercised (1,2). This happens for a variety of reasons, including the reloading of energy substrate, the repair of micro damage to utilized muscle groups and may also be influenced by the activation of the sympathetic nervous system. This metabolic boost, in my opinion, is the real benefit of cardiovascular training.

There are 3 basic components to a cardiovascular exercise program that need to be addressed: 1) Type 2) Frequency/Duration and 3) Intensity.

Note

Before we get started, I recommend that you mention to your doctor that you are starting an exercise program and want to make sure you are medically cleared to do so. This is very important and often I will not recommend any exercise for a new client until I receive medical clearance. I will be asking you to work at a moderate to high intensity with regards to heart rate and it's important that you have the confidence that it is safe to do so. Now let's break down the 3 parts of the cardio program.

Type

The type of cardiovascular exercise you engage in is entirely up to you. Let your individual preferences guide you. However, do realize that some exercises will be more effective in helping you to achieve your goal of lasting weight loss.

Best Choices
Walking or Walk/Jog Intervals
Elliptical Trainer
Stair Climber

Secondary Choices
Bike
Roller Blading
Ice Skating
Swimming
Jogging
Aerobic Dance

You can see the types of cardio are broken down into Best Choices and Secondary Choices. As the name implies, the Best Choice exercises will be your main source of cardio; the one you'll do the most consistently. These exercises are typically easy to learn, are not weight supported and therefore force you to work harder and expend more calories. These choices also provide minimal impact on your joints.

Elliptical Trainer

I am sure you have seen these machines on television or at the gym. God bless the man or woman who invented the elliptical trainer! It truly gives you the best of both worlds. You get the calorie burning potential of a more strenuous method of cardio, like running, but with very low impact. There is minimal stress on your joints when using this machine. The movement is very fluid, and a lot of fun. I feel like I'm working as hard as I do when I run but feel none of the impact. This is usually my first choice of cardio if my clients can get access to one of these machines. Just about every gym has elliptical trainers and there are now lower costing models for the home. The Gazelle Sprintmaster is under $200, give this one a try!

Walking or Walking/Jogging Intervals

If you are 30 or more pounds overweight or older than 50, you may want to start with walking as your source of cardio. To start with, walking is easy, we all know how to do it. Walking is also convenient. Weather permitting, you can just head outside any time you want. Walking is inexpensive, a good pair of running or walking sneakers is all you will need. All in all, walking is a great way to get started. After a while, walking will no longer be intense enough for you to continue losing weight. At this time, you may want to graduate to a walk/jog interval training program. With this type of program, you jog for 2 minutes and then walk for 3 minutes and repeat this throughout the cardio session. You will get the benefit of burning more calories than walking without the continual high impact on your joints associated with running.

Once you hit the point where walking is no longer intense enough (you'll know it's time when the scale stops moving downward) you can continue to utilize walking as your main cardio choice but you'll have to greatly increase your time commitment. At this point, I'll give my clients one minute toward their cardio goal for every 2 they walk. So, if your goal for cardio is 200 minutes a week, you will need to walk 400 minutes.

Stair Climber

The stair climber is also a great form of cardio that qualifies for the Best Choice group. These have been around for years and do a good job of burning calories while keeping the impact on your joints to a minimum.

Secondary Forms Of Cardio

The secondary forms of cardio either require a lot of skill, have an increased risk of injury, are expensive or inconvenient for one reason or another. These modes of cardio are fine for a substitute now and again (once or twice a week) but I wouldn't recommend them to be done on a consistent basis.

Bike Riding

There are 2 types of bike riding. Riding outdoors on the street can be dangerous and is highly dependent on the weather. Riding indoor on a stationary bike is safe and independent of the weather, but in both cases, the bike is supporting your weight, so you burn far fewer calories than you would with a primary form of exercise. Now and again this is OK but certainly not as your major source of cardio. If you absolutely love to bike or spin, you can count 1 minute toward your cardio goal for every 2 minutes you bike or spin.

Rollerblading

This is a great, lower impact form of cardio that burns tons of calories and is loads of fun. I'm a hockey player and love skating in all of its forms. The reason why it is not on the primary list is that it takes a fair amount of skill, carries with it a significant risk of injury and is highly dependent on the weather. The same goes for ice skating.

Swimming

Swimming is a great form of exercise. You work every muscle in your body. It's on the secondary list for several reasons. Not many people can get to a pool multiple times a week, so there is the issue of accessibility. Furthermore, since the water is supporting your weight, you're not burning as many calories as you would with an upright form of exercise, like elliptical training. Swimming is also very difficult from a fitness standpoint. Most people simply can't swim long enough to hit their cardio minute goals.

Jogging

I normally do not recommend jogging as a method of cardio to my clients. When we run, we can put up to 6 times our body weight on our joints. I weigh 180 pounds, so when I run, I am putting the equivalent of 1,100 pounds on my joints. I don't think that we were designed to do this for long periods of time. Just about every client that I've had that insists on running for their major source of cardio will, over time, sustain an overuse injury that keeps them on the sideline at some point and usually repeatedly. It's a shame too, because you burn a lot of calories when you run.

If they really want to run, I advise my clients to engage in an interval type training. I have them run for 2 minutes and then walk for 3 minutes and repeat. This gives you the best of both worlds; you get an increased calorie burn from the jogging without the chronic stress on the joints.

Aerobic/Group Exercise Classes

Aerobic classes can be an effective source of cardio but there are usually a few problems with them. Often, they are high impact and tough on the joints. Furthermore, these classes are usually stop and go with regards to heart rate and I'm generally looking for a more consistent heart rate demand. If your aerobics class is easy on the joints and you truly are working hard the whole time, then this can be your main source of cardio. If not, limit yourself to one or two classes a week and pick a primary source of cardio.

Group exercise classes with weights have become popular recently. While these classes are great, when it comes to weight loss, I generally like to have my clients separate their cardio and weight training. The goal of resistance training is to build muscle, while the goal of cardio is to elevate heart rate and burn calories. It is difficult to accomplish both of these activities in one session. To optimize weight loss, I recommend that you do them separately.

Frequency And Duration

There are a lot of opinions about the optimal frequency and duration of cardio sessions for the weight loss client. Some trainers feel that you should work out every day, others say that you should work out in the morning and still others suggest splitting the workout into several smaller sessions throughout the day. While there are merits to each of these theories, I have found that in practice, the only really important factor is total minutes of cardio per week. I give my clients a certain number of minutes that need to get done and it is entirely up to them how they do it. I care about the intensity and the total minutes, that is all.

What The Research Tells Us

The research literature has shown us just how much cardio is necessary to successfully lose weight and keep it off. Let's take a look at some of the more influential investigations.

A great place to start is The National Weight Control Registry. The NWCR is an ongoing study established in 1994 by collaborators from Brown Medical School and the University of Colorado (3). This study is the largest prospective investigation of long-term successful weight loss and weight maintenance. To enter this study, participants have to prove a weight loss of at least 30 pounds that has been kept off for a minimum of 1 year. Over 4,000 subjects are being tracked and the average weight loss is 72 pounds kept off for over 5 years. This is a very impressive amount of weight loss and more importantly, maintenance of weight loss. The researchers periodically publish results describing how these people have maintained their weight loss. The average physical activity of these successful losers is equivalent to 1 hour a day of brisk walking.

A similar result was found in the Women's Health Study. This is a prospective investigation of just under 40,000 women out of Harvard University. In 15 years of follow-up, the only women that did not gain weight as they aged were those that engaged in cardiovascular exercise for 60 minutes per day (4).

In an 8-year follow-up of the Nurses' Health Study II cohort, only 38% of the women avoided weight gain during the study. They averaged 36 minutes per day of physical activity (5).

The research literature also shows us that cardio-vascular exercise is really important to maintain lost weight. After a 29 lbs. weight loss, 82 women were ran-domized to a group that was instructed to walk 2-3 hours per week, a group that was instructed to walk 3-6 hours per week or a control group (6). By the end of 40 weeks, the control group had regained 4½ pounds back, while the exercise groups lost an additional 1½ pounds. This is a 6-pound swing in less than a year.

In the Nurses' Health Study II cohort, 4,558 subjects who had reported a recent weight loss of 5% of their body weight were followed for 6 years of weight maintenance (7). Compared to women who were seden-tary, women who exercised for at least 30 minutes per day were significantly less likely to regain 30% or more of their lost weight.

It is abundantly clear that exercise needs to be a big priority if weight loss is your goal. Again, I really don't care how you break it up, as long as you get the minutes. A common number of cardio minutes that I'd give to a male weight loss client is 150 minutes a week. I don't care if he does 6 times a week for 25 minutes, 4 times a week for 38 minutes or 3 times a week for 50 minutes. The truth of the matter is that it doesn't affect the results too much either way. However he can fit it into his life is fine by me. I care only that the minutes are done consistently.

The number of cardio minutes you will need to lose weight is highly subjective and will change as you progress toward a more healthy weight. If you have a lot of weight to lose, many pounds will come off with lower levels of cardio. Eventually, more cardio will become necessary to keep the scale moving in the right direction. Having said this, here is a general recommendation:

Women

I must say that when it comes to weight loss, I do feel a little bit sorry for the ladies. Because men have more muscle than women, they have a much easier time losing weight and can get away with far lower levels of cardio. But you know what they say: "That which we obtain too easily, we esteem too lightly". In my experience, most women will lose the vast majority of their weight getting 250 minutes of cardio a week. That is 36 minutes a day, 7 days a week or 42 minutes a day, 6 days a week or 50 minutes a day, 5 days a week. I know that this sounds like a lot, and it is, but it is absolutely necessary.

Don't jump right into this amount. Work your way up to it. If you are really out of shape or deconditioned, start with 120 minutes the first week then progress to 175 minutes in week 2 and then hit the 250 by week 3.

If you hit a plateau that lasts 2 weeks or longer and your diet has been good and you've done your resistance training religiously and you've followed the lifestyle guidelines, you may want to increase your cardio by 10-

20 minutes a week to get the scale moving again. In most cases, 250 minutes is all you'll need. The maximum cardio you should do is 300-350 minutes per week. If you do more than this, you run the risk of breaking down muscle tissue for energy which will hurt you in the long run by decreasing your metabolism. Another problem with too much cardio is that it can increase your appetite, which will lead to overeating.

If you hit this maximum level and your weight is still not where you want it to be, cardio is not the problem. Look into your diet, lifestyle habits or resistance program and chances are one of these facets of the program are slowing you down.

Men

Men get off easy when it comes to cardio. Usually 150-180 minutes is all that will be needed. As with the ladies, if you are out of shape or deconditioned, go easy at first. Start with 75 minutes the first week then progress to 120 minutes the second week and then progress to the full 150 by the third week.

If you hit a plateau that lasts 2 weeks or longer and your diet has been very good and you've done your resistance training religiously and you've followed the lifestyle guidelines, you may want to increase your cardio by 10-20 minutes a week to get the scale moving again. However, in most cases, 150-180 minutes is all you'll need.

Intensity

The intensity of your cardiovascular program is very important. If you are not working at the proper level of intensity, your rate of weight loss can really slow down.

Generally, you want to work just below your anaerobic lactate threshold, which is between 70-85% of your maximum heart rate. You may have heard of people taking their heart rate or calculating their target heart rate zone to gauge intensity. Well, I'm not going to ask you to do that. #1) It is complicated. #2) The maximum heart rate formulas do not apply to a large segment of the population. #3) There are easier ways.

There are a few simple strategies to ensure that your intensity is where it needs to be:

1. *Are you sweating?* After about 5 minutes into your workout, you should be starting to sweat. If you are not, then you have to pick up the pace. You don't need to be dripping sweat to satisfy this test, but you should notice some sweat at least under your armpits. Not the most pleasant test, but it works.

2. *Can you talk?* Another simple way to gauge intensity is the talk test. In the middle of your workout, try talking to someone (or yourself if need be). If you are taking a breath after every 2 words, you're working too hard and need to slow down. If you are able to string multiple sentences together without stopping for air, you need to pick it up. You should be able to say a normal length sentence without taking a breath. But you should need to take a breath after this sentence.

3. *Ratings of perceived exertion.* When you are working out, stop and ask yourself: "How hard am I working on a scale from 1 to 10?" On the following page you can see a sample rating of perceived exertion scale with descriptions for

each level. The level of 7 and 8 corresponds with both the sweating and the talk test. Shoot for that.

Level 10---All out maximal sprint. You could last at this level for maybe 30 seconds.

Level 9---Close to maximal effort. You could last a few minutes at this pace.

Level 8--- Sweat test/talk test

Level 7--- Sweat test/talk test

Level 6---Walking very fast. As if you're late for an appointment.

Level 5---Walking moderately fast

Level 4---Walking normally

Level 3---Walking at a slow pace

Level 2---Standing still

Level 1---Sitting down and reading

Here are some more tips to help you keep your intensity in the ideal range:

1) When using a machine like the elliptical trainer or stair climber, keep the resistance very low and move quickly. When the resistance is set too high, your leg

muscles can tire and prevent you from getting the aerobic minutes you need.

2) When using an elliptical trainer, ignore the arms and just use your legs. I want the focus of the work to be on the large muscle groups of the lower body, and not on the arms.

3) As your fitness level begins to rise, you can add some interval training to your cardio routine. Here's how to do it: Start your cardio at your normal pace. After 4½ minutes, increase your speed for 30 seconds. Wear a watch and time this. You don't need to go all out, just increase your speed a bit. After the 30 seconds are over, return to your normal level of cardio for the next 4½ minutes. Repeat these interval sprints 4 times during your cardio session. This is a great way to boost your calorie burn. I generally reserve interval training for my younger and healthier clients. If a client is very overweight or has risk factors for heart disease (high blood pressure, high cholesterol, insulin resistance), I don't recommend interval training, as the increased intensity can spike heart rate and blood pressure.

Additional Benefits Of Cardio

Imagine if a new medication was introduced to the market that helped you lose weight. Imagine if this medicine also decreased the risk of heart disease, stroke, diabetes, cancer and Alzheimer's disease. Imagine if it would also reduce blood pressure, improve blood cholesterol profiles, increase your energy and reduce both anxiety and depression. This drug would also combat insomnia, improve your sex drive and actually increase your confidence and self-esteem. Sounds like a dream, right? Too good to be true?

This last paragraph pretty much sums up the many benefits of cardiovascular exercise. If a drug like this actually came to market, I bet in 2 months 90% of the adult US population would have a prescription for it.

The research literature shows us just how important cardiovascular exercise is to our health. Very large and well-designed studies have shown that those who exercise regularly have a reduced risk of heart disease (8), stroke (9), diabetes (10), certain cancers (11,12), cognitive decline (13) and all-cause mortality (14,15).

Amazingly, according to the Centers For Disease Control, only 51.7% of Americans attain the recommended levels of physical activity to provide these health benefits. And only 21.7% met the goals for both cardiovascular exercise and strength training activity (16). What a shame.

Tips For Getting Your Cardio Done

I've been working with clients who want to lose weight for well over 20 years. I know that it is not easy to fit cardio into your busy life. However, it is important to keep in mind that unless you hit your cardio minutes consistently, there is very little chance that you will attain your weight loss goals.

In general, the most cardio I ever have a client do is 45 minutes, 5 to 6 times a week. Trust me, I know this is a time commitment, but you must work on making it a priority. Getting this cardio done consistently will improve just about every area of your life; your health, your energy, your mood, even your self-esteem. You get a lot back from this investment. So, here are some tips to help you get cardio into your life on a consistent basis.

#1) *Make it a priority.* First of all, consciously understand the importance of getting your cardio done for your health and weight loss goals. Exercise really is one of the most important things on your daily to do list. Don't be so quick to blow it off.

#2) *Keep a record of your daily cardio minutes.* Write your minutes of cardio in a journal, add them up each week and see how well you did. There is something about seeing things in black and white that helps us to be more accountable. This can also be a tool to adjust your program. Look for patterns. Maybe you'll see that Monday is so busy that you keep missing your cardio; make sure that is one of your days off.

It's important to have the right frame of mind when keeping cardio logs. Don't expect them to be perfect. Don't beat yourself up if your log is not exactly as it should be. We all slip up with our diet and exercise, that's human nature (even I do!). See the log for what it is; a valuable tool to help you track your highs and lows and your overall progress. Don't feel like you're being graded here.

#3) *Consider getting a piece of cardiovascular equipment for your home.* I always advise my clients to get some type of cardio equipment in their home. There are several reasons why this is critical. If you are doing cardio 5 or 6 times a week, it can be difficult if not impossible to get to the gym all of those days. If you have a piece of equipment at home, you can hop on for 15 minutes here and 20 minutes there and get the job done. It also takes the weather out of the equation if you are currently exercising outdoors.

There is no need to get a very expensive machine. There are a number of home models that are reasonably priced. I currently recommend the Gazelle Sprintmaster to my clients. This is an in-home elliptical trainer that costs under $200. When I lived in apartments in Boston, I had one myself and loved it. Now if you want to invest a little more money, Life Fitness sells home models that are virtually identical to their gym quality elliptical machines. I have one of these now and absolutely love it.

Consider it an investment in your health and your future. If you took one year's worth of gym dues, you'd be surprised at how nicely you can make a little gym in your home. A piece of cardio equipment, a simple flat bench and some dumbbells will cost less than many gym's yearly dues and last a lifetime, or close to it. Remember, we need consistency above all else. Make it easy for yourself by working out at home.

#4) *Killing 2 birds with 1 stone.* Try to combine your cardio with something you already do every day. Let me tell you a little story. Several years back I had a client named Beverly who was trying to lose weight. Beverly had the diet down very well and I was working with her twice a week in her home lifting weights, so her resistance training program was dead on. She was a very busy women working as a school teacher and had many family obligations. She just couldn't get her cardio in and this fact was greatly slowing down her results.

I let her know that her inability to get the requisite cardio was slowing her progress. She said she really wanted to get it done, but she just couldn't seem to fit it in. I asked her about her daily schedule. After work got out, she'd rush home to start preparing dinner or baby sit her grandson or one of a million other things. She also mentioned that she always watched her favorite TV show, "Who Wants To Be A Millionaire", with her husband. Bingo! I said to her "Hey Beverly, why don't you put a TV in front of your treadmill and get your cardio done as you watch the show?". Well that was the trick. Beverly never missed that show and after this small adjustment, she never missed her cardio either. She quickly hit her goal weight and when I left her, she was on a nice maintenance program.

Look at your daily schedule. Is there something that you do every day for 30 or 40 minutes that you could combine with your cardio? Is there a TV show that you watch, maybe the news? You can easily read on most pieces of cardio today, why not combine your daily look at the newspaper with your cardio. I've been known to return phone calls and even study while doing cardio when my schedule becomes particularly busy. Having a piece of cardio equipment in your home makes it surprisingly easy to hit your goal for the week.

#5) *Distraction.* At the end of the day, some people just will never like doing their cardio, and that is OK. For these people, distraction is the key. Listening to music, a podcast or a book on tape can make the time go by much quicker. If you have a cardio machine at home, putting a TV with a DVR in front of it can be a real game changer. There have been times that I have been watching a really good movie while working out and have completely forgotten that I was even doing cardio.

The bottom line is that if you make your cardio a priority, you can find a way to fit it in. "I'm too busy" is not a good excuse. Ironically, it is usually my most busy clients that find ways to get their cardio done because it becomes a priority to them when they realize they must do it to reach their goals. Make it a priority for you, too!

ACTION STEPS FOR THIS CHAPTER

1. Talk to your doctor and get clearance before starting any new exercise program.
2. Pick a "Primary" source of cardio for most of your work. These exercises will facilitate more efficient weight loss.
3. Get your minutes in each week. In general, women will need 250 and men will need 150.
4. Work at the proper intensity. Remember "The Talk Test", "The Sweat Test" and "The Ratings Of Perceived Exertion".
5. Keep a record of your cardio minutes and add them up each week to help you stay on course.
6. Consider getting an inexpensive piece of cardio equipment for your home. This will make it much easier to be consistent with your exercise.

Chapter 8

Resistance Training

Resistance training, also known as weight training, is the last but certainly not least component of your weight loss program. More often than not, it is completely ignored by those trying to lose weight. A lot of misconceptions about resistance training are part of the reason why this is so. Let's start from the beginning-Why is resistance training so vital to the weight loss effort?

The human body can broadly be broken down into 2 components: fat mass and lean body mass. Fat mass is rather self-explanatory; it's your body fat. Lean body mass is basically everything else; your bones, muscles, organs, connective tissue, etc. There are lots of differences between the functions of fat and lean body mass. That is not really within the scope of this chapter. What you need to know is that lean body mass burns calories and fat does not.

Lean Body Mass Burns Calories And Fat Mass Does Not

Muscle is a constantly changing tissue. It needs to be supplied with energy, it needs to be repaired and rebuilt after minor trauma. Fat, as you can imagine, is not really all that active. It just kind of hangs out there and stays put. It would make sense that the more muscle you have, the more calories you will burn each day in an effort to maintain it. This means that you will burn more of the calories that you ingest and less will be stored as fat. This is a major benefit of resistance training.

As part of the aging process, we start to lose muscle as we enter adulthood. This begins around the age of 30 and gradually progresses so that in our 50's we are losing 1-2% of our muscle each and every year (1). Every pound of muscle burns roughly 6 calories a day (2). Therefore, if you lose 5 pounds of muscle as you enter your mid to late thirties that would be 5 x 6 = 30 calories every day that you once burned but are now storing as body fat. Thirty calories a day really does not sound like much, but trust me, this adds up. In a year's time, 30 calories per day is equivalent to over 3 pounds gained in a year. This is a primary reason why people gain weight as they age, even if their total calorie intake does not increase at all!

With resistance training, you can counter this loss of lean tissue and even increase your muscle mass. In some ways, resistance training is like the fountain of youth. It can roll back the hands of time with regards to your metabolism and lean body mass.

It's also important to realize that when you lose weight without resistance training, you lose both muscle and body fat. This is the body's defense mechanism to prevent its fat stores from dropping too low, too fast. After all, we evolved in times of famine and food scarcity. If your fat stores got too low and you hit a famine, that would be the end of you. When you lose weight without strength training, the amount of muscle lost can reach a significant percentage of lost weight. There has been some interesting research on this topic.

Ninety-four overweight women were randomized to one of 3 groups while losing 25 lbs. (3). One group lifted weights, one group engaged in cardiovascular exercise and the other was a control. The control subjects who did not lift weights lost over three pounds of muscle, which was 12% of weight lost. The resistance exercise group lost no muscle, they actually gained a pound of lean body mass as they lost their weight.

In a similar study, 40 women were randomized to one of 4 groups for an 8-week weight loss study (4). One of these groups was a diet only group and another was a diet and strength training group. In the diet only group, 20% of the weight they lost was muscle. In the resistance trained group, only 12% of lost weight was lean body mass.

In another trial, 65 men and women were randomized to diet only, diet plus strength training or diet plus aerobic exercise groups for an 8-week weight loss study (5). In the diet only group, 28% of the weight they lost was muscle. In the resistance training group, only 8% of lost weight came from muscle.

There is evidence that this preservation of lean body mass has a favorable impact on resting metabolic rate. In the study mentioned three paragraphs above, the researchers also measured resting metabolic rate. In this investigation, 94 subjects were randomized to 3 different groups while losing 25 pounds: a cardio group, a strength group and a control group (3). By the end of follow up, the control group had a 103 calorie per day decrease in resting metabolic rate. The aerobic exercisers had a 76 calorie decrease. The weight lifters had only a 44 calorie per day decrease. Compared to the control group, the weight lifters had a 59 calorie per day advantage, which over the course of a year equates to more than 6 pounds worth of calories burned.

It is clear that when you add resistance training to your weight loss plan, you lose a significantly higher amount of fat and a significantly lower amount of muscle, which helps result in permanent weight loss.

Some people avoid resistance training because they fear they will bulk up and become muscle bound. I have found this to be a particular concern of my female clients. First of all, it is not easy to bulk up. Body builders spend a lot of time lifting heavy weights in a highly organized program designed to build muscle. The type of weight training program that I advocate here is to enhance weight loss and general health and fitness, the goal is not to build large amounts of muscle. You will notice increased strength and muscle definition for sure but not large increases in muscle mass. You will be using lighter weights and higher repetitions to help build lean, toned physiques. Women also don't need to worry about bulking up because they generally lack the levels of testosterone necessary for that type of growth.

Resistance training is not just for those looking to lose weight; it is important for every single adult. Losing muscle and strength really impacts our ability to function as we get older. In fact, a lot of what we associate with aging really is just the loss of strength. So, starting a weight training program will not only help you lose weight and keep it off, it will set you up for an active and healthy life in your later years.

Frequency And Sample Programs

How many days a week do you need to lift weights? A minimum of 2 and a maximum of 3. It is important to not workout with weights two days in a row. The body needs rest to repair the muscles you use. Therefore, workout on non-consecutive days such as Monday, Wednesday, Friday or Tuesday, Thursday and Saturday. Now I will provide a sample program for men and for women. These are programs designed to enhance weight loss and they can be done quickly; in about 20-30 minutes. Each of these exercises will be illustrated in the next chapter.

Sample Programs

Men

Bench Press	3 sets of 7-10
1-Arm Row	3 sets of 7-10
Front Raise	3 sets of 7-10
Bicep Curl	3 sets of 7-10
1-Handed Overhead Press	3 sets of 7-10
Standing Squats	3 sets of 7-10
Abdominal Crunches	3 sets of 7-10

Women

Assisted Squats	3 sets of 8-14
Inner Thigh Lifts	35- 50 (each side)
Standing Side Raise	15-25 (each side)
Bench Press	3 sets of 8-14
1-Arm Row	3 sets of 8-14
Front Raise	3 sets of 8-14
Bicep Curl	3 sets of 8-14
Kick back	3 sets of 8-14
Abdominal Crunches	3 sets of 10-20

Why is the men's program different than the women's? Most of the men I've trained have the goal of adding a little muscle mass in addition to losing weight. For this reason, the repetitions for their exercises are a little lower and the weights that they use to perform their exercises are significantly higher. This will help them attain their goals. Most of the women I've trained are not at all interested in building large amounts of muscle, they just want to tone up and look tighter. The program for women reflects these goals.

What Weights Should I Use?

This is a very difficult question to address in a book because each person is starting at a different level of strength and fitness when I first meet them. I've roughly broken it down into 3 classes and then given examples of starting weights. Remember, this is a rough estimate. Your weights will depend on your own subjective view of how hard you are working. Similar to the cardiovascular training guidelines, on a scale from 1 to 10 you should feel like a 7 or 8 on your last set. This is not a maximal effort but no stroll through the park either!

Men Beginner*

Bench Press	8 lbs. dumbbells
1-Arm Row	8 lbs. dumbbell
Front Raise	5 lbs. dumbbells
Bicep Curl	8 lbs. dumbbells
1-Handed Overhead Press	5 lbs. dumbbell
Standing Squats	Body Weight

Start with these weights if you have never lifted weights before.

Men Intermediate*

Bench Press	15-20 lbs. dumbbells
1-Arm Row	15-20 lbs. dumbbell
Front Raise	8-10 lbs. dumbbells
Bicep Curl	15 lbs. dumbbells
1-Handed Overhead Press	8 lbs. dumbbell
Standing Squats	10 lbs. dumbbells

Start with these weights if you have some experience with these exercises and weight training in general but have not been lifting consistently.

Men Advanced*

Bench Press	25-30 lbs. dumbbells
1-Arm Row	25-30 lbs. dumbbell
Front Raise	12-15 lbs. dumbbells
Bicep Curl	20 lbs. dumbbells
1-Handed Overhead Press	10-12 lbs. dumbbell
Standing Squats	15-20 lbs. dumbbells

Start with these weights if you have been lifting consistently for 2 years or more. These weights may seem low, I'll explain later.

Female Beginner*

Squats	Assisted
Inner Thigh Lift	Body Weight
Standing Side Raise	Body Weight
Bench Press	5 lbs. dumbbells
1-Arm Row	5 lbs. dumbbell
Front Raise	3 lbs. dumbbells
Bicep Curl	5 lbs. dumbbells
Triceps Kickback	5 lbs. dumbbell

Start with these weights if you have never lifted weights before.

Female Intermediate*

Squats	Body Weight
Inner Thigh Lift	Body Weight
Standing Side Raise	Body Weight
Bench Press	8 lbs. dumbbells
1-Arm Row	8 lbs. dumbbell
Front Raise	5 lbs. dumbbells
Bicep Curl	8 lbs. dumbbells
Triceps Kickback	8 lbs. dumbbell

Start with these weights if you have been lifting for a few months but inconsistently.

Female Advanced*

Squats	5-8 lbs. dumbbells
Inner Thigh Lift	Body Weight
Standing Side Raise	Body Weight
Bench Press	10 lbs. dumbbells
1-Arm Row	10 lbs. dumbbell
Front Raise	6-8 lbs. dumbbells
Bicep Curl	10 lbs. dumbbells
Triceps Kickback	10 lbs. dumbbell

Start with theses weights if you have been lifting consistently for 12 months or more.

Why Are These Weights So Low?

This is a program that is designed to enhance weight loss. It is not designed to build large amounts of muscle or strength. Remember, 50% of your weight loss results will come from dietary change, 30% from cardiovascular exercise and 20% from resistance training. Since most people are really busy and don't have unlimited time to devote to their fitness, these programs cover the basics for resistance training in the shortest time possible. By all means, if you have the time and interest and prefer a more detailed weight training program feel free! But for the goal of weight loss, more extensive programs are not really necessary.

Perform the program with 25 seconds rest in between sets and no rest in between exercises. Wear a watch and time this! There are two ways to get a response from your muscles. You can use heavy weights and take long rests (optimal for body building and higher levels of strength and muscle mass) or you can use lighter weights with shorter rests (optimal for toning and weight loss). I choose the latter for my clients because: 1) They don't have much time and working out this way speeds up the workout. 2) In my experience, lighter weights decrease the risk of injury. Here is an example of a sequence of exercises with the appropriate rest intervals:

Bench Press 1st Set Of 8

--25 Second Rest--

2nd Set Of 8

--25 Second Rest--

3rd Set Of 8

--No Rest--

1-Arm Row 1st Set Of 8

--25 Second Rest--

2nd Set Of 8

--25 Second Rest--

3rd Set Of 8

--No Rest--

Front Raise 1st Set Of 8

--25 Second Rest--

Etc

I would recommend that if at all possible, you do your resistance training at home. Invest in a simple bench and some adjustable dumbbells. Women can buy individual sets of dumbbells; 3lbs., 5lbs. and 8lbs. are all you'll need. Men can pick up adjustable dumbbells. A set that can take you from 5-30 pounds should do it. You may want to purchase an inexpensive flat bench to help with some of the weight exercises. This equipment won't cost you much and the routines will typically take only 20-30 minutes to do. This is probably less time than it takes to drive to and from the gym and change your clothes.

What About Progression?

For women, whatever level you are, start the weight exercises with 3 sets of 8 repetitions. Slowly increase to 3 sets of 14 repetitions. When this becomes less of a challenge, increase your weight by a few pounds and drop back down to 3 sets of 8. This is called a double progression program.

It is the same idea for men but start at 3 sets of 7 and work your way up to 3 sets of 10. When this becomes easy, increase the weights by a few pounds and drop back down to 3 sets of 7 repetitions. Take your time increasing your repetitions and weights, this is not a race. Only increase a few repetitions per week.

Your muscles will begin to get used to the challenges that these exercises present and will ultimately stop reacting and growing. For this reason, after 6-8 weeks, it's a good idea to switch up your exercises in order to keep your muscles guessing. For men, switch to the following program:

Chest Fly
Overhead Press
Military Press
Concentration Curls
Triceps Kickbacks
Lunges

Here is a second program for women as well:

Plie Squats
Standing Inner Thigh Lifts
Side V's
Chest Fly
Overhead Press
Military Press
Hammer Curls
Overhead Triceps Press

Most of these exercises are really basic. However, if you feel intimidated or unsure, consider hiring a personal trainer for a session or two. It's a great investment to ensure that you are doing the exercises properly. I recommend that you hire a trainer with a degree in exercise science and at least one nationally recognized certification such as ACE (The American Council on Exercise) or ACSM (The American College of Sports Medicine).

There are two keys to a successful strength program. The first is consistency; you need to hit the weights regularly. The second is variability. In order to confuse your muscles, you need to switch up your exercises every 6 weeks. Remember, although not as important as your diet and your cardio, it is absolutely essential that you fit in at least two and preferably three 20-30 minute weight training sessions a week in order to hit your weight loss goals.

ACTION STEPS FOR THIS CHAPTER

1. Realize the critically important role of resistance training in attaining your goal of lasting weight loss.
2. Hit the weights at least twice a week, preferably 3 times a week.
3. Slowly increase your repetitions and your weights. You don't want to simply repeat the same workout over and over. You need to keep your muscles guessing.
4. For the same reason, switch your exercises every 6-8 weeks.
5. If all this seems too intimidating, consider hiring a personal trainer for a session or 2 to get you started.
6. If at all possible, pick up some dumbbells and do your training at home. It will be much easier to fit it in if you don't have to go to the gym to do it.

Chapter 9: *Guide To Resistance Training Exercises*

Bench Press

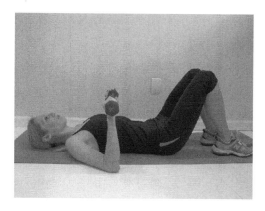

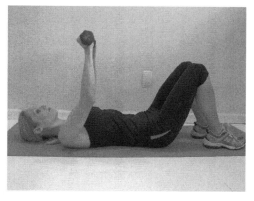

Targets: Chest and Triceps
1. Lie on bench or floor (bend knees if on floor).
2. Hold dumbbells at the sides of your chest along the line of your sternum.
3. Lift dumbbells toward the ceiling.*
4. Slowly return to starting position.

*With this exercise and all others, exhale during the active phase of the exercise, when you are working against gravity. Inhale when you are working with gravity in the passive phase of the exercise. Don't hold your breath! Holding your breath may cause your blood pressure to rise to a dangerous level.

1-Arm Row

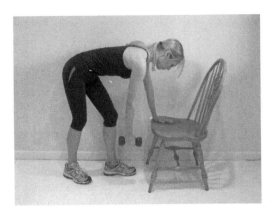

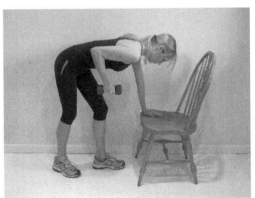

Targets: Back
1. With your left arm on a bench or chair, hold a dumbbell in your right hand.
2. Let your arm hang directly down in front of your shoulder.
3. Slowly pull the dumbbell up toward your chest.
4. Slowly lower the dumbbell to starting position.
5. Keep your back flat and centered over the bench. Your elbow should be tight against your ribcage as you lift and lower the dumbbell.
6. Alternate sets between your right and left hand.

Front Raise

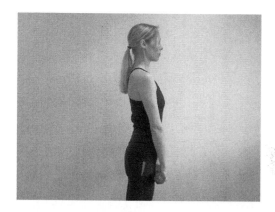

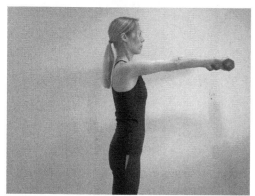

Targets: Shoulders
1. Stand up straight with your feet shoulder width apart and your knees slightly bent.
2. Hold dumbbells directly in front of you with your palms facing your thighs.
3. Slowly raise dumbbells to shoulder level (no higher).
4. Slowly lower to starting position.

Bicep Curl

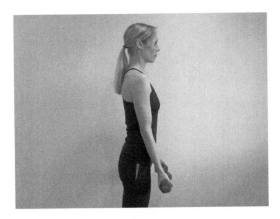

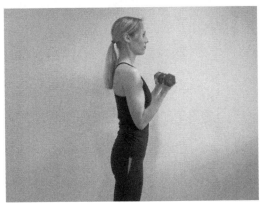

Targets: Biceps
1. Stand with your feet shoulder width apart and your knees slightly bent.
2. Hold dumbbells with your arms at your sides and your palms facing forward.
3. Keep your shoulders still and slowly bend your elbows to raise dumbbells by just moving your forearms.
4. Slowly return to starting position.

1-Handed Overhead Triceps Press

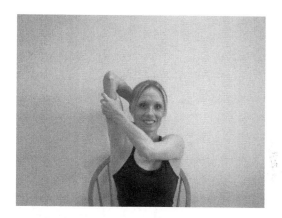

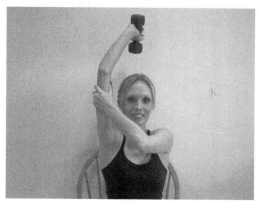

Targets: Triceps
1. Grasp a dumbbell with your right hand behind your head with your elbow bent.
2. Keep your upper arm fixed from shoulder to elbow.
3. Raise the dumbbell toward the ceiling until your arm is straight.
4. Slowly return to starting position.
5. Alternate sets with right and left hand.

Standing Squats

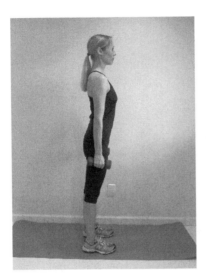 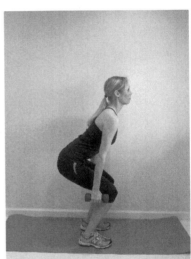

Targets: Legs
1. Stand upright with your feet shoulder width apart.
2. Hold dumbbells at your sides.
3. Bend your knees until your thighs are almost parallel to the ground.
4. Slowly return to starting position.
5. Don't let your knees cross the plane of your toes.

Abdominal Crunches

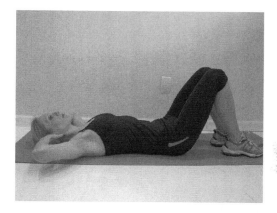

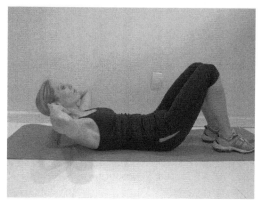

Targets: Stomach (abdominals)
1. Lie on your back with your knees bent and your feet flat on the ground.
2. Put your hands behind your head with your elbows pointing outward.
3. Curl your body upward toward your thighs until your trunk reaches a 45° angle with the floor.
4. Slowly lower to starting position.
5. Keep your feet on the floor at all times.

Assisted Squats

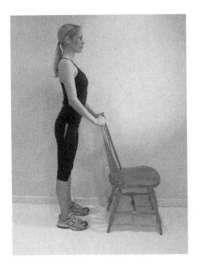 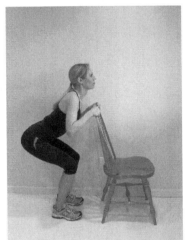

Targets: Legs

1. Stand in front of a pole or a sturdy chair with your feet shoulder width apart.
2. Slowly bend your knees until your thighs are almost parallel to the floor.
3. Hold onto a pole or chair for balance only. Don't use the chair to pull yourself up. Your weight should be on your feet so your legs do the work.
4. Slowly rise to starting position.
5. Make sure your knees don't cross the plane of your toes. This puts unnecessary strain on your knee joint.
6. If you find this exercise too difficult, start out with a Sit Squat. Actually sit in the chair with your hands on your thighs and stand up. Sit back down and repeat for the desired number of reps.

Inner Thigh Lift

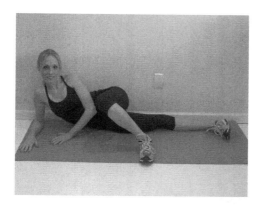

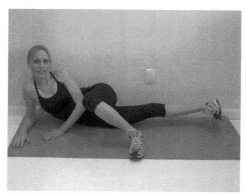

Targets: Inside of thigh
1. Lay on your right side with your right leg straight and your left leg bent over your right leg.
2. Keeping your right leg completely straight, raise it up toward the ceiling.
3. Slowly lower to starting position.
4. Repeat on your left side.

Standing Side Raise

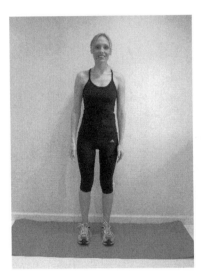 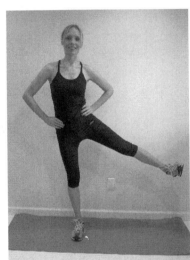

Targets: Outer thigh
1. Stand up straight and lean your right hand against a wall or pole for balance, if necessary.
2. Raise your left leg until it is nearly parallel to the floor.
3. Slowly return to starting position.
4. Alternate sets between your left and right legs.

Triceps Kickback

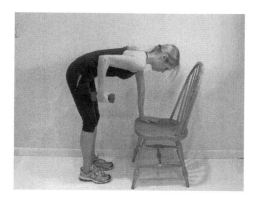

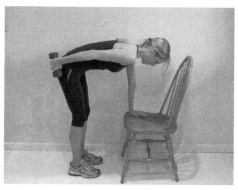

Targets: Triceps
1. Hold a dumbbell in your right hand.
2. Bend at your waist and rest your left hand on a bench or chair.
3. Your back should be parallel to the floor.
4. Raise your elbow up to the level of your ribcage and keep your arm close to your body.
5. Extend the dumbbell back until your arm is straight, keeping your upper arm motionless. Only your forearm should be moving.
6. Slowly return to starting position.
7. Alternate sets between your left and right arm.

Chest Fly

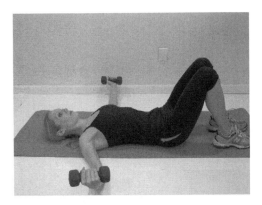

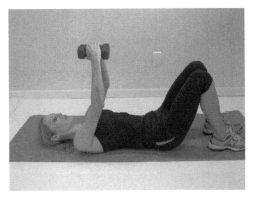

Targets: Chest
1. Lie on floor or a bench (bend knees if on floor).
2. Grasp a pair of dumbbells and hold them above your chest with your palms facing one another.
3. With elbows slightly bent, lower your arms until they are slightly above your shoulders.
4. Keep the weights in line with your breast bone.
5. Slowly return to starting position.

Overhead Press

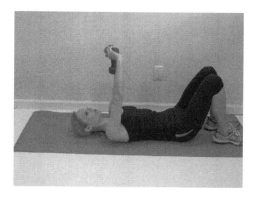

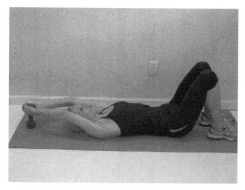

Targets: Back
1. Lie on floor or bench (bend knees if on floor).
2. Hold a dumbbell between your thumb and forefinger of both hands letting it lay perpendicularly above your chest.
3. With your arms straight, extend the dumbbell behind your head until it almost reaches the bench or floor.
4. Slowly bring back to starting position.

Military Press

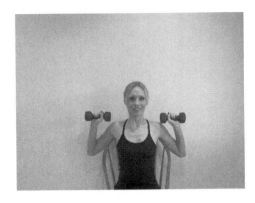

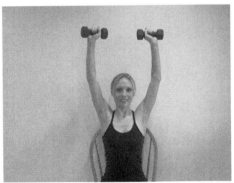

Targets: Shoulder
1. Sit on a chair or bench with your feet flat on the floor.
2. Hold dumbbells at shoulder height with your palms facing forward.
3. Raise the dumbbells toward the ceiling keeping them lined up with your ears.
4. Slowly lower the dumbbells back to starting position.

Concentration Curls

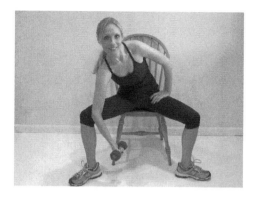

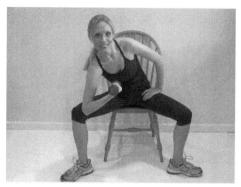

Targets: Biceps
1. Sit on a chair or bench with your legs spread wide apart.
2. Hold a dumbbell with your arm pressed against your inner thigh.
3. Curl the weight up toward your chin.
4. Slowly lower to starting position.
5. Alternate sets between your right and left side.

Lunge

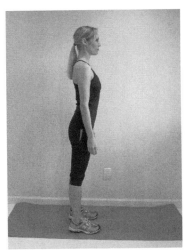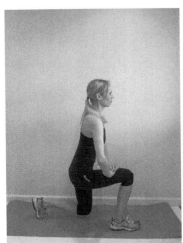

Targets: Legs
1. Stand with your feet shoulder width apart.
2. Slowly step forward with your right leg and drop your left knee almost to the ground. Rest your hands on your right thigh.
3. Make sure your knee does not cross the plane of your toes.
4. Slowly return to starting position.
5. Alternate sets between your right and left leg.

Plie Squats

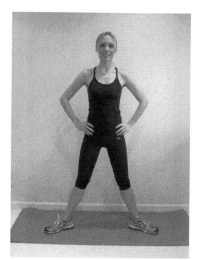 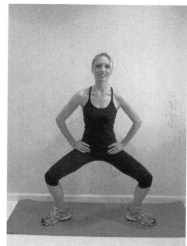

Targets: Legs
1. Stand with your feet spread widely apart and your toes pointing outward.
2. Bend down at the knee until your thighs are almost parallel to the floor.
3. Slowly return to starting position.

Standing Inner Thigh Lifts

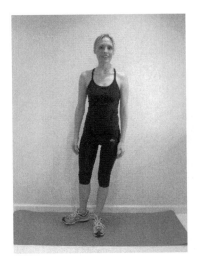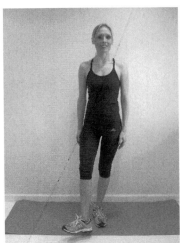

Targets: Inner thigh
1. Stand up straight and lean against a pole or wall for balance, if necessary.
2. Point the toes of your right foot outward so you form a right angle with your left foot.
3. Move leg forward 1-2 feet.
4. Slowly return to starting position.
5. Alternate sets between both legs.

Side V's

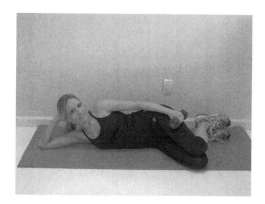

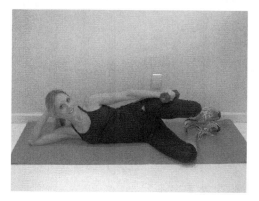

Targets: Outer thigh
1. Lay down on your right side with your knees bent and your feet together.
2. Hold a dumbbell on your left thigh midway between your knee and hip.
3. Slowly open your legs apart, keeping your feet together at all times.
4. Slowly return to starting position.
5. Alternate sets between both legs.

Hammer Curls

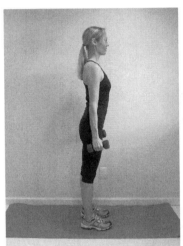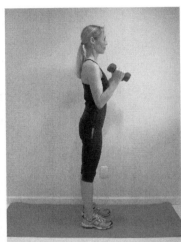

Targets: Biceps
1. Stand with your feet shoulder width apart and knees slightly bent.
2. Hold dumbbells with your arms at your sides and your palms facing one another.
3. Keep shoulders still and slowly bend your elbows to raise dumbbells by just moving your forearm.
4. Slowly return to starting position.

Chapter 10

Lifestyle Factors

So far, we have very effectively covered the big 3 components of this weight loss program: diet, cardio and resistance training. Now it is time to focus on lifestyle and behavioral factors that will go a long way in helping along the weight loss process.

#1 Write Down What You Eat And Your Daily Cardio Minutes.

Keeping a record of your diet and cardio is a valuable tool to help you gauge your progress. It is also accountability! Knowing that you have to answer to someone, even if it is yourself, helps you to make better choices consistently.

In fact, I attended an obesity symposium at Harvard Medical School a few years back where a researcher there told an interesting story. This particular scientist had designed a study to examine the effects of 2 different diets on weight loss, a low-fat diet and a low carbohydrate diet. The idea was to randomize the subjects into 2 groups, one group would follow the low-fat diet and the other would follow the low-carb diet for several months and then the amount of weight lost would be compared between the 2 groups. In an effort to make sure that the 2 groups were similar in their baseline diets prior to entering the study, the participants were told to simply write down everything that they ate for a period of 2 weeks. They were instructed to not change anything about their diet, just to write it down. Would you believe that every single participant lost weight in these 2 weeks, by doing nothing more than writing down what they ate?

I have my clients write down what they eat for at least a few weeks. It is invaluable for giving them a sense of control over their food selections. It sounds like an inconvenience, but in actuality it takes just 30 seconds after each meal; just 1½ minutes a day to greatly help you toward your weight loss goal. Well worth the investment! Again, this won't need to go on forever, but do it for the first few weeks. A simple pocket-sized memo book is all you will need. Just write the date on top of the page and then fill in your carbohydrate, fat and protein selection for breakfast, lunch and dinner. You don't even have to write down your portions, just what you ate. See the sample on the following page. You can even keep track of your food intake on your smartphone with any number of apps that are free to download. Two really good ones are *My Fitness Pal* and *Lose it.*

It's equally important to document your cardio-vascular exercise. How else will you be able to tell with certainty if you have hit your weekly goal of cardio minutes? Furthermore, if you have a week or two where your weight loss has slowed, it is very easy to see which part of your program was responsible for the plateau if you've kept records of your diet and cardio.

Date: Monday July 18th   **Cardio**: 45 minutes

Breakfast: Protein: Low-fat plain yogurt
Carbohydrate: Strawberries
Fat: Peanut butter

Lunch: Protein: Tuna fish
Carbohydrate: Salad vegetables
Fat: Olive oil and vinegar

Dinner: Protein: Chicken breast
Carbohydrate: Brown rice, vegetable stir-fry
Fat: Canola oil used in stir fry

#2 No Eating After 8:00 PM

This is a really important lifestyle change if you want to be successful in the weight loss game. While the research is generally lacking in this area, there are a couple of studies utilizing weaker designs that suggest a relationship between late night eating and weight gain. Anecdotally, I have noticed that this is a really important lifestyle factor for my clients. If they consistently eat after 8 PM, they really don't lose much weight. When they stop eating after 8, they do lose weight. Let's take a quick look at the research evidence.

In a recent cross-sectional investigation published in the *American Journal of Clinical Nutrition,* 110 college-aged men and women recorded all of their food intake with a time stamp so that the hour of consumption could be accurately recorded. When compared to normal weight subjects, overweight subjects consumed significantly more of their calories 1 hour closer to melatonin onset, which was around 11 PM (1).

Another cross-sectional investigation published in the journal *Appetite* showed that protein, fat and carbohydrate consumed after 8:00 PM were associated with a higher BMI in a group of 52 volunteers that filled out 7-day food logs (2).

There are several reasons why eating food after 8 PM increases the risk of weight gain:

-Eating food late at night simply adds extra calories that you would not consume otherwise.

-Food consumed late at night is usually of poor nutritional quality and more likely to cause weight gain. Most people snack on high glycemic carbs like chips, pretzels and desserts late at night. We have learned in previous chapters how these blood sugar spiking foods promote weight gain.

-Another hypothesis is that our metabolism slows down quite a bit at night, so more of what we consume is stored as fat.

-The thermic effect of food may be lower at night, so more of what we eat is stored as fat. In fact, an older study showed that 9 young men burned a higher percentage of a standardized meal's calories in the morning and afternoon than they did at night (3).

I have had clients who were exercising well and did a nice job following the diet but lost little weight until they implemented this rule. I can add a little story from my own personal experience. Growing up, I had the exact opposite problem that my clients hire me to help them solve. I could not gain weight for the life of me. You could count my ribs- I was that skinny. I was tired of looking so emaciated as I got into high school and started eating all the time. Nothing happened! I got a job at a bake shop and literally ate bread, cookies and anything else for 5 or 6 hours after school. Unbelievably, I still would not gain a pound. My metabolism just seemed to burn up whatever I threw at it.

I graduated high school and went off to college as thin as ever. A fraternity brother told me that one of his buddies back home had the same problem and he finally gained weight by eating 2 peanut butter sandwiches right before bed. Well I tried it. I ate 2 peanut butter and jelly sandwiches right before I went to bed every night of the summer between freshman and sophomore years in college. I gained an astonishing 30 lbs. in 4 months! I tell you this story to make the following point: if eating food late at night finally put weight on a young kid with a super high metabolism, what will it do to an older individual with a slower metabolism? You guessed it, nothing good.

Do your very best with this one. I know it can be difficult. People are in the habit of making dinner reservations at 8 or 9 PM on the weekends. This must change. Make your reservations a little earlier. Have dinner first on your own and then meet up socially for a movie or something else. You need to learn that your lifestyle habits are the major reason why you have gained weight in the first place. If you don't change them, you'll be stuck in the same situation for sure.

One last note: most of my clients can get away with eating after 8 one night per week. I, myself, almost always eat after 8 PM on Saturday nights. However, if it happens more often than this, late night eating can really hurt your chances of hitting your goal weight.

#3 Drink 8 Glasses Of Water A Day

Everyone who is interested in losing weight has heard this one a million times. It is not just an old wives' tale. There is evidence in the research literature that drinking water helps along the weight loss process. Let's take a quick look at some of these studies.

-In a combined analysis of Harvard's Nurses' Health Study, Nurses' Health Study II and Health Professional Follow-up Study that included almost 125,000 subjects followed for approximately 20 years, each cup of water consumed per day was associated with a modest weight loss (4).

-Forty-eight adults were assigned to one of two diet groups for 12 weeks (5). The first group was assigned a low-calorie diet. The second was assigned the same diet, but was instructed to drink 16 oz. of water right before each meal. At the end of the 12 weeks, the group drinking the water prior to each meal lost an additional 4.5 pounds.

-The Stanford University A to Z weight loss trial also examined water intake and weight loss (6). This trial was designed to compare the weight loss efficacy of 4 popular diets over a year in 173 young women. In a secondary analysis, they found that women who drank more than a liter of water each day (a little more than 4 cups) lost an additional 5 lbs. after a year.

There are several potential reasons why drinking water helps along the weight loss process:

-*Increased metabolic rate.* Drinking water appears to increase sympathetic nervous system activity, which increases metabolism. Calories are also utilized to warm the water to body temperature. In the research literature, drinking 16 oz of water increased metabolic rate 30% in normal weight subjects (7) and 24% in overweight subjects (8).

- *Gastric distension.* Water may also increase gastric distension, which has the potential to decrease hunger and subsequent energy intake. Fifty subjects participated in a trial that compared energy intake after consuming a water preload (9). All subjects had access to an all you can eat lunch both with and without drinking 16 oz. of water 30 minutes before the meal. Energy consumption at the lunches were compared. The subjects over 60 years of age consumed a statistically significant 58 fewer calories after drinking the water preload. Interestingly, this was not seen in the younger subjects.

- Water replaces beverages containing calories. If you are drinking a lot of water, then you are probably not drinking a lot of soda or juice. The elimination of these calories over time can positively impact weight. In the earlier mentioned study that combined 3 Harvard cohorts, replacing a cup of sugar sweetened beverage with a cup of water resulted in over 3 and a half times as much weight loss as drinking water alone (4).

A couple of notes on the water intake. Do your very best to sip water throughout the day instead of chugging 2 or 3 glasses at once when you realize you're behind on your water requirement. This is to avoid having to run to the bathroom often. It goes without saying that any beverage that contains added sugar should be avoided. Soda, fruit juice, sports drinks and energy drinks are not the way to go if your goal is adequate hydration.

Caffeine is an interesting question. The research has gone back and forth on whether caffeinated beverages are as effective at hydrating our body as caffeine free choices. In large doses, caffeine can act as a diuretic. I am confident saying that a cup of caffeinated coffee or tea a day is not a problem. However, I always tell my clients that the majority of their beverages should be caffeine free. When it comes to hydration, I'd stick with old fashioned water, decaf tea and coffee and my personal favorite, flavored club soda.

Most of us walk around dehydrated all the time and don't even know it. When you are well hydrated, you'll feel better and have more energy. Do your best to hit 8 glasses of water each day.

Specifics On Beverages
Water- The best!
Fruit Juices-No Good; Sugar
Diet Soda-No Good; Caffeine
Coffee/Tea-No Good; Caffeine
Club Soda/Sparkling Water-Good!
Decaf Coffee/Tea-Good! (But Don't Add Sugar)
Sports drinks-No Good; Sugar
Energy drinks-No Good; Sugar

#4 Limit Your Consumption Of Alcohol

Alcohol has become an area of great interest in the fields of nutrition and medicine in recent years. Too much alcohol is like poison to the body causing a variety of negative health effects such as liver disorders, cancer and vitamin deficiency as seen in alcoholics. However, a moderate amount of alcohol (1-2 drinks a day) appears to decrease the risk of heart disease, stroke, and diabetes as well as increase overall longevity.

These two facts have put doctors and nutritionists in a difficult position regarding alcohol recommendations. On the one hand, we don't want to push alcohol use and risk alcoholism in those genetically prone to this terrible disorder. Yet the potential health benefits of moderate alcohol use are difficult to ignore. I hate to complicate matters further, but here goes:

If you want to lose weight, strictly limit alcohol use. The research tends to go back and forth on this issue, but there is definitely evidence that supports a relationship between alcohol consumption and weight gain (10-13).

Let's take a look at one of the better designed studies in detail. Researchers from Harvard combined subjects from 3 separate cohorts into a giant study on individual foods and weight gain (10). Over 120,000 men and women were followed for up to 20 years. Increases in alcohol, even just one drink a day, were significantly and consistently associated with modest weight gain. There are several reasons why this may be true:

-Alcohol is calorie dense, it contains 7 calories per gram and these are nutritionally empty calories that provide little besides energy. A typical beer has 150 calories, a glass of wine has 85 calories and 1.5 ounces of hard liquor generally has 100 calories. Have 2 or 3 of these a day and trust me, the calories begin to add up. Furthermore, liquid calories generally don't register with the body. In other words, if you eat a solid food snack right before dinner, you would compensate by eating a little less at dinner. The body does not seem to recognize liquid calories in the same way. So, if you have a drink or two before dinner, you don't eat any less food. In this way, alcohol calories are simply added on rather than substituted.

-Alcohol can't be stored in the body, so it becomes a priority for oxidation. Because of this fact, alcohol consumption suppresses fat oxidation. Therefore, you are burning less of your body fat when you drink.

-In my experience and that of my clients, when you have a few drinks and start to get a bit of a buzz, your discipline goes out the window. When you drink, inhibitions of all types are lessened. You begin to think "Why not, you only live once". This causes many otherwise bright people to make bad decisions! After 3 or 4 drinks, the dessert menu becomes harder to resist and the late-night fast food/diner stop seems to become all but inevitable! Alcohol is thought to impair satiety and activate food reward signaling. In an interesting study, 1,864 men and women were selected from the National Health and Nutrition Examination Survey who reported drinking alcohol on one of their 24 hour recalls but not on the other (14). When drinking alcoholic beverages, the men consumed an additional 168 non-alcohol calories with increases in saturated fat, sodium, meat and potatoes. Women consumed 93 more calories per day when they drank, consuming a higher saturated fat content.

You don't necessarily have to give up alcohol here. If you have a few drinks a week, say four or less, you'll be fine. If you're drinking every day, this can really slow your rate of weight loss. A good strategy that several of my successful clients have used is to drink only on the weekends and avoid alcohol completely during the week.

#5 Limit Sugar Free Sweeteners

As you have probably noticed, the increase in the prevalence of type 2 diabetes and the popularity of low carbohydrate diets has created a gigantic market for sugar free products. It is now common to see sugar free ice cream, cookies, candies, pies and protein bars in addition to the all familiar diet soda. It makes sense that people trying to eliminate sugar from their diet would be interested in these types of products.

The first question I usually get about non-nutritive sweeteners is if they are safe to consume. The idea that non-nutritive sweeteners are cancer causing chemicals from hell is pretty common thanks to the internet. However, in reality, they are well tested and overall very safe to consume, particularly when used in moderation.

Well-designed studies show that moderate non-nutritive sweetener use is not associated with weight gain (15), heart disease (16), type 2 diabetes (17), stroke (18) or cancer (19).

Just because sugar free products are generally safe to consume does not mean you have the green light to have as much as you want of them. For people trying to lose weight, there are a few problems with non-nutritive sweeteners that leads me to recommend limiting their use to just a few times per week.

The first problem I have found is they do tend to perpetuate your cravings for sugar. If you get sugar out of your diet, in about 2-3 weeks you won't miss it or crave it at all. If you consistently consume these sugar free products, the cravings never really go away entirely and you'll always be fighting them to one degree or another. This is a problem because any diet where there is a continuing feeling of deprivation will not result in long term weight loss.

Another issue I have found with daily use of non-nutritive sweeteners is that they can make you more hungry in general, which is certainly no help to someone trying to lose weight. There is research to back this up. In an interesting randomized crossover trial, 12 subjects had glucose, fructose or the non-nutritive sweetener acesulfame-K injected directly into their stomach on separate occasions (20). Hunger and satiety were measured by means of visual analogue scales. There was a statistically significant steeper return of hunger and decrease of satiety after the non-nutritive sweetener than after glucose or fructose.

In another interesting trial, 12 subjects consumed both sugar and artificial sweetener on separate occasions while undergoing a brain MRI (21). Different parts of the brain responded when the subjects consumed the non-nutritive sweetener than when they consumed sugar. Without getting too technical about the specifics of this complex study, the researchers believed that the non-nutritive sweetener activated taste reward circuits, but did not satisfy the subjects in the same way as the sugar. This leaves the door open for an increase in hunger after consumption of the non-nutritive sweetener.

Another potential problem with the non-nutritive sweeteners deals with something called the cephalic response. If you were to put your favorite food in front of yourself, your eyes would see it, your nose would smell it and your body anticipates you are about to eat it. There is evidence that your body releases digestive enzymes in anticipation of the meal before you even put it in your mouth! The same may be happening with the non-nutritive sweeteners. The body thinks it's getting sugar when you eat these and may release insulin in response.

A recently published randomized trial provides some evidence that this may be the case. A group of 33 subjects consumed a high dose of non-nutritive sweet-ener (over 10-13 packets per day) for 14 days (21). Four separate measures of insulin and glucose sensitivity were taken at the end of follow-up. Compared to a control group, subjects consuming the non-nutritive sweeteners had a significantly lower insulin sensitivity by the end of follow-up. There was no difference in the other 3 measures of insulin or glucose efficiency.

In summary, moderate consumption of sugar free products is really not a problem for your health or your weight loss goals. However, going overboard with these products may make it much harder to lose weight. Limit yourself to just a couple servings of these products each week. In just a bit, we'll cover when it's best to add them into your diet.

#6 Shoot For At Least 7 Hours Of Sleep Each Night

There is strong evidence that sleep deprivation increases risk of weight gain (10,23). There are several proposed mechanisms.

Sleep deprivation may increase energy intake: In a randomized crossover trial, 30 men and women were studied under both short sleep duration (4 hours per night) and long sleep duration (9 hours per night) for 5 nights (24). On the 5th day, they were given unlimited access to food and consumption was closely monitored. When subjects were sleep deprived, they consumed 295 more calories per day than when they had a full night's sleep.

Sleep deprivation may decrease metabolic rate: In a randomized crossover trial, 14 normal weight men had their energy expenditure measured by indirect calorimetry on two separate occasions; after 8 hours of sleep and after complete sleep deprivation (25). When compared to a normal night's sleep, energy expenditure was reduced by 5% following sleep deprivation.

Sleep deprivation may decrease diet quality: In another interesting trial, 42 short sleepers (5 to less than 7 hours per night) were randomized to either a sleep extension or control group (26). The sleep extension group received behavioral training designed to increase sleep duration. After 4 weeks, the sleep extension group increased their sleep by 47 minutes per night. After adding this sleep, the extension group reduced their added sugar consumption by 2½ teaspoons per day compared to the control group.

There are several potential explanations for these findings. Sleep deprivation appears to lower leptin, a hormone that influences metabolism and satiety. Sleep deprivation also appears to raise ghrelin, a hormone produced in the stomach that increases hunger. Sleep deprivation may alter neuronal pathways that regulate reward behaviors. Finally, being fatigued from a lack of sleep may reduce physical activity. Even though we are not totally sure why sleep deprivation increases weight, it sure seems to be important. Do your best to get at least 7 hours of sleep each night.

#7 Splurge Meals (AKA Planned Relapses)

No diet needs to be 100% perfect in order to attain your weight loss and health goals. I've asked you to change your diet dramatically and to give up foods that you were eating every day and love to eat. Total deprivation of these foods is neither realistic nor necessary. If your diet is tight 90% of the time, you will hit your weight loss goals for sure. That means that 10% of the time you can have some fun. Since we eat 3 meals a day for 7 days a week, that's 21 meals per week and 10% of 21 is approximately 2. So, for 2 meals a week you can basically ignore everything I've told you about diet and eat exactly what you want. I call these splurge meals or planned relapses.

Did you really think that I'd ask you to give up bread, pasta and dessert forever? We both know that's not going to work. If I did, you'd probably hang in there for a few weeks, maybe even a few months but eventually you'd break down and have something from the avoid column and say, "This guy is crazy, I can't do this anymore" and pretty much quit. I call these splurge meals a planned relapse because you have total control over them. You plan when you have them and you stop after 2 a week and there is no guilt because you've done nothing wrong. You don't even have to write what you ate in your food log. Just write "Splurge Meal".

If you're smart, you'll plan one of these splurge meals on Wednesday and the other one on Saturday, so you never have to go more than 3 days without one of your favorite foods you're trying to cut back on. Be creative, if it's pizza that you miss the most, have that. If it's a cheeseburger, then go for it! No guilt, no worries. Plan your splurge meals in advance. If you know you'll be having dinner at a wedding or party, don't even try to be good, make it a splurge meal and have fun with it. The key is you are in total control.

There are only two rules to follow when it comes to splurge meals: The first is to stay away from sugar. If you have sugar even twice a week, there is a really good chance you will start to want it all the time. The reason this dietary plan works so well is that after a couple of weeks, there really is no deprivation. Once your blood sugar stabilizes, you won't crave bread, pasta, rice and sugar much at all. If you are constantly battling cravings for sugar, it will be very hard to stay focused. It sounds unbelievable but it's true: It is easier to give up sugar 100% than 75%.

However, we all like something sweet now and again. There is currently a huge assortment of sugar free treats available. You can find sugar free chocolate, peanut butter cups, ice cream, cookies and even cupcakes. Feel free to enjoy some sugar free treats during or after your splurge meals. They are made with non-nutritive sweeteners and sugar alcohols. Start slowly with them because the sugar alcohols can have a laxative effect in sensitive people and that's no fun for anyone. In the next chapter, I will list a bunch of the best sugar free treats I have tried and where to find them.

The other rule to follow when splurging is to avoid back to back splurge days. It is really important to bracket a splurge meal with a couple of days of good eating on either side. This helps to stabilize your blood sugar and will keep carb cravings from creeping back in.

The best schedule for my clients seems to be a Wednesday night and a Saturday night splurge, but it is certainly up to you to find what works best for your life.

ACTION STEPS FOR THIS CHAPTER

1. Keep a log of your diet and cardio minutes.
2. Strictly limit eating after 8:00 PM.
3. Drink 8 glasses of water each day.
4. Keep alcohol containing drinks to 4 or less per week during the weight loss phase.
5. Limit non-nutritive sweeteners to a couple of times a week.
6. Try to get at least 7 hours of sleep each night.
7. Plan 2 splurge meals a week. Feel free to eat anything you want during these meals except for sugar. If you want something sweet after a splurge meal, grab a sugar free treat.

Chapter 11

Final Thoughts and Frequently Asked Questions

OK, so you've finished the book. I've thrown a lot at you and I'm sure your head is spinning! You should feel optimistic because you are about to make some great changes that will positively influence just about every aspect of your life. Congrats for taking the first important step.

One last piece of advice: slow and steady wins the race. Very few people can just adopt all of these lifestyle changes right away. Some get their cardio and diet down but have trouble with the weight training. Maybe getting the cardio in will be your greatest challenge.

The weight loss process has a lot of ups and downs, good weeks and bad weeks. The key to success lies in picking yourself up when you fall down. Persistence is the key to weight loss but remember, this is not rocket science. This program works and you can make it work for you. Keep in mind that I've just given you the "gold standard" for weight loss, everything you can do to lose weight effectively and permanently. You'll also lose weight on the "silver" or "bronze" standard, but just a bit more slowly. In other words, if you are only able to do ¾ of what I'm asking you to do, you'll still get results, it will just take you a bit longer to hit your goals.

Over the years I have observed 2 traits that predict success on this program. The first one is to plan ahead. Do your grocery shopping early in the week and have everything you need ready to go. If you have the right proteins, fats and carbs in stock you will always be able to throw together a healthy meal no matter what life throws at you. Similarly, planning ahead is important for your splurge meals. Take a look at your week and use your splurge meals for those times that you won't be able to control your food.

The other really important trait is resiliency. I've got a newsflash for you: you will make mistakes following this program. There will be all sorts of screw ups, especially early on. I know that I sure had plenty of them as I began to adopt these diet and exercise habits. You need to have a real short memory and get right back on track after you mess up.

My two favorite sports are football and hockey. In football, the most important position is quarterback. When a great quarterback throws an interception, he basically forgets that it happened. He goes out on the very next drive with the same confidence he had before he threw the pick.

The same is true of a great hockey goaltender. Every goalie lets in a soft goal now and again. The good ones shake it off immediately and forget about it. That is how I want you to be with your diet. If you miss an exercise session or have an extra splurge meal, shake it off and get right back in the game. Don't beat yourself up. I have found that clients who possess this quality have a much better chance of attaining their goals.

I'd like to finish off this chapter with questions that I have been frequently asked by my clients and readers of my other books over the years.

How fast will I lose weight?

You need to understand that a pound of fat is a lot of calories, 3,500 in fact. To lose one pound of fat in a week, you'd have to create a caloric deficit of 500 calories every day. That is either eat 500 fewer calories or exercise away 500 calories. This is easier said than done.

We live in a world where people expect fast results. You can get a meal at a fast food restaurant in 2 minutes. You get money from an ATM instantaneously. Our bodies don't work quite the same way. For my male clients, a good average weight loss is 1 pound a week. Women have it a bit tougher, ¾ of a pound a week on average is great. Three-quarters of a pound a week may not sound like much but that's 36 pounds in a year and will result in permanent weight loss since we are sparing lean tissue. Remember to always look to the average. You may lose a lot of weight in one week, lose nothing in the next week and then even gain a pound in the following week. Always look at the average. As long as you are at or above ¾ of a pound a week, the program is working.

There is evidence that when you lose a lot of weight very quickly, the body fights hard to put it back on. A gentler and more gradual weight loss is easier for the body to accept. That should be your goal. One other tip: Don't get too wrapped up on weight. Remember, you are adding muscle while you are losing fat. The scale will reflect this. For the majority of my clients, the very best measure of their progress is not the scale but how their clothes are fitting them.

How often should I weigh myself?

I suggest that you weigh yourself one time a week, the same day every week, first thing in the morning without any clothes on and before you eat or drink anything. Make sure at least 2 days have passed since your last splurge meal before you weigh yourself. The reason for this is that consuming extra salt, alcohol or white flour can cause you to retain a few pounds of water for a couple of days. Ladies, also keep in mind that during that time of the month you can also retain a few pounds of water so don't freak out if the scale goes up a bit around this time every month.

Most of my clients splurge mid-week on Wednesday and once on the weekend. Therefore, I recommend you pick either Wednesday morning or Saturday morning for your weigh in. This ensures that you'll get those 2 days of clean eating before your measurement.

I am a big fan of Tanita scales and have been using and recommending them for years. These are research quality scales that are very accurate, but not too pricey. I personally have a Tanita Ironman model that also allows me to take my body fat. You can pick these up at amazon.com and learn more about them at Tanita.com.

Do you have a list of foods I should always keep stocked?

In order to set yourself up for success, your home has to become your oasis for healthy eating. This means doing your own grocery shopping, and cooking your meals the vast majority of the time. Here are the top 15 food items to always keep in your pantry or refrigerator. If you have these tried and true, nutrient packed foods ready to go, you are never more than a few minutes away from a healthy, blood sugar stabilizing meal.

#1 Vegetables: Variety is the key here, and the more the merrier. Include vegetables for salads, sweet potatoes, broccoli, cauliflower, spinach, and on and on.

#2 Fruits: Again, variety is the key. Make sure to get a bunch of fruits that travel well, such as apples and oranges. You can throw these in a backpack or purse and they are always ready for you no matter what your day brings.

#3 Nuts: An excellent source of healthy fat that travels well.

#4 Nut Butters: Peanut butter, almond butter, cashew butter, macadamia nut butter, pistachio butter. They are all really good.

#5 Olive Oil: Great for salad dressing and to sauté vegetables.

#6 Old Fashioned Slow Cooked Oatmeal: A nice lower glycemic whole grain packed with fiber. Don't get instant or quick cooking as these are higher glycemic. Focus on the "Old Fashioned" slow cooking variety.

#7 Black Beans: Great in a salad or even on their own. These are an excellent source of low glycemic carbo-hydrate and vegetable protein loaded with fiber,

vitamins, and minerals. Try to find a low sodium version.

#8 Quinoa: An awesome whole grain that is high in fiber and protein.

#9 Tuna Pouches: These are relatively new. They are tuna fish in a pouch that you simply tear open and eat. You don't need to drain this tuna or use a can opener. Highly portable, these are great on the road or even on an airplane.

#10 Chicken Breast: Buy in bulk at Costco or BJ's and keep in your freezer.

#11 Eggs: An excellent source of both fat and protein. They take about 5 minutes to prepare when cooking them and even less if you hard boil them ahead of time and have them ready to go.

#12 Olivio or Smart Balance: These are butter substitutes made from olive and canola oil. You can use these any time you'd use butter. They taste really good and are so much better for you than butter.

#13 Brown Rice: A great lower glycemic whole grain that is a good source of cereal fiber. Make sure you get the slow cooked variety and not instant or quick cooking as these are higher glycemic.

#14 Sliced Turkey Breast: A low fat, convenient source of protein. Try to get it freshly sliced off a bird and not the pre-packaged variety that is filled with nitrates and

preservatives. Fully cooked rotisserie chickens are a similarly good choice.

#15 Frozen Shrimp: A delicious source of protein that is surprisingly reasonable when bought frozen in bulk at Costco or BJ's.

Do you have any tips on how to stay on track when I am eating out at a restaurant?

One thing that you always need to keep in mind about restaurants is that they are businesses. Like all businesses, their primary objective is to make money. They do not have your health as their primary goal. They are not thinking about your weight loss goals. Their main objective is getting you back in their restaurant again and again and again. They accomplish this goal by making their food taste great. In general, restaurant food has an overabundance of:

- Calories
- Fat
- Saturated Fat
- Sugar
- Salt

Here are a few tips to help guide you through the treacherous waters of dining out:

1) Don't eat out as much as you do right now. It sounds simple. It is simple. Eat out less. When you shop and prepare your own food, you are in complete control of what you eat. In restaurants, you are hopelessly out of control and at the mercy of the chef. Remember, the chef's primary goal is to improve the taste of the dish, not improve your health. Do your grocery shopping once a week, and get enough food to prepare the lion's share of your meals at home. It may be an obvious strategy, but it is the most important one.

2) Use your splurge meals strategically. You have two meals a week to go off the plan and eat whatever you want, except for sugar. If you know you'll be eating out, use one of these splurge meals, and you won't have to worry about being perfect. Splurge meals are great when you can't control your food 100%. Saving them for when you eat out is a great strategy to stay on top of your game.

3) Do some online menu research. Almost all restaurants now have their menus online. Check them out. Come up with a list of restaurants in your area where you can eat clean, and another list for the "splurge only" spots.

4) Don't be afraid to ask for what you want. Most restaurants are more than happy to substitute menu items if you ask. When I'm at a restaurant that I'm not too familiar with, I'll scan all the menu selections to see what side dishes are available. I recently was at a restaurant that had a healthy grilled fish dish that came with a potato side. I noticed that a steak dish came with sautéed spinach. I ordered the fish, but asked to substitute the spinach for the potato. The chef was more than happy to do so.

5) Some specific guidelines:
*Start with a protein. Just about every restaurant will have a variety of proteins to choose from. Look for options that don't have a lot of sauces, such as grilled chicken, lean steak, fish or other seafood.

*Shoot for vegetables for your carbs. This includes salads, sautéed vegetables or sweet potatoes. If the restaurant offers whole grains like brown rice or quinoa, feel free to add one of these as well.

*Use healthy vegetable oils to round out your fat serving. Ask for olive oil and vinegar on the side when ordering a salad, or ask that your vegetables be sautéed in olive or canola oil.

*Limit sauces and dressings that are creamy or sweet. Always get your sauce or dressing on the side, and put a reasonable amount on your dish. A good guideline is to put half of what they give you on your food.

*When the server brings bread, kindly refuse it. If service is on the slow side and you're hungry, seeing warm bread and butter may be too much for you!

*If possible, substitute brown rice for white rice. Many restaurants can now accommodate this request.

*If a dish comes with pasta, white rice, or potatoes, ask for sautéed vegetables or a side salad instead.

*In general, stay away from prepared salad dressings. They are usually too high in saturated fat and/or sugar. Instead, ask for olive oil and vinegar on the side. This way you can control your fat portion completely.

6) *Be an early bird.* Eating out and eating late seem to go hand in hand. This is a 1–2 punch combination to your waistline that is difficult to defend. Do your best to make reservations as early as possible. Remember that you need to be done eating by 8:00 PM. When you absolutely can't control the time of your reservation (at a business meeting, for example), eat before you go and get a small salad or bowl of soup for your entrée. I've had clients in the past successfully use this strategy.

Do you have any tips on how to stay on track when I am traveling?

Traveling presents some unique challenges for those trying to lose weight. Here are some of the major issues:

- We are in far less control of our food.

- It is more difficult to exercise.

- We tend to drink more alcohol.

- Our sleep is often disrupted.

- A "vacation mentality" lends to a more carefree attitude regarding our diet and exercise.

- We eat out every meal. This has a negative impact on our calorie, fat, salt, and sugar intake.

I think of travel as falling into two separate categories. The first is vacation travel. This type of travel happens for most of us only once a year, and will last for about a week on average. The second type of travel is more frequent work-related travel. For a number of my clients, work related travel amounts to 50% of their year. Each type of travel requires a distinct strategy, and therefore, we will deal with each separately.

Vacation

Here are some tips to help you deal with vacation travel. Once again, this type of travel is of short duration and happens infrequently, usually only once a year for most of us.

1) Adjust Your Goals. Here's a statement that may surprise you: you are not going to lose weight on vacation so don't even try to. Your goal for vacation is weight maintenance, but in all likelihood, you'll gain a few pounds. If you go away for only one week a year, I expect and even want you to have some fun. You'll probably eat a bit more and drink a bit more, and the truth of the matter is that you should, it's your vacation! Go away with the attitude that you'll try to maintain your weight or even gain a pound or two. Any weight that you add will come off quickly once you get back and resume your healthy lifestyle. The truth of the matter is that you simply can't do that much damage in one week, especially if you follow these tips.

2) Maintain Your Exercise To Minimize The Damage. I don't recommend cutting back on your exercise during vacation. Get your daily cardio, and hit the weights a few times during the week. It should be easier to find time to exercise on vacation than any other time of the year. In fact, when I go away, exercise is really the only thing on my to do list. I will not even think about booking a trip to a hotel or resort without gym facilities.

3) Eat Conservatively For Breakfast And Lunch, Splurge A Bit On Dinner. Eat a healthy breakfast and lunch as you normally would at home. Feel free to splurge a bit on dinner. This ensures that you will be eating sensibly most of the time, but will allow you to eat for fun each day of your vacation as well.

4) Stay Away From Sugar, Even On Your Vacation. Sugar is unique in its ability to completely derail your diet. I've seen it dozens of times. If you have sugar even once, you start to want it again. Then you have it again, and want it some more. After a few days of this, other refined carbs like bread, pasta, white rice, and potatoes become irresistible to you.

The solution is to just stay away from sugar, even when on vacation. Feel free to enjoy a sugar free dessert if it is available. I know that most cruise ships now serve a variety of sugar free desserts. In time, I'm confident we'll see more and more sugar free offerings at restaurants and resorts. However, if you don't think they will be available, bring some sugar free cookies along with you on vacation and eat them for dessert. Avoid sugar at all times and at all costs.

5) Prepare For Increased Cravings When You Return Home From Your Vacation. After splurging a bit more on your vacation, carb cravings will likely return with a vengeance. Prepare for them mentally. Also prepare for them by having all of your healthy foods stocked and ready as soon as you get back. A trip to the grocery store immediately upon your return is a necessity. After a few days you should be fine, particularly if you avoided sugar.

<u>More Frequent Work Related Travel</u>
If you travel often for work, a different strategy is necessary. You cannot allow yourself to get into a situation where you blow off your diet and exercise every time you are on a trip. You've got to learn to function on the road as you would at home. This is difficult, but not impossible. It is all about preparation, planning ahead, and keeping your diet and exercise goals a priority when you are away. Following are a few tips for the more frequent business traveler.

1) If At All Possible, Travel Less. If you are at all able to control your travel schedule, do everything you can to minimize the number of trips or the length of your trips. I do understand that this is not a possibility for a great number of business travelers. However, if you are self-employed or in control of your travel schedule, this is a great place to start.

2) Keep Exercise On Your Schedule While Away. Just because you are away for a few days doesn't mean that you can blow off your exercise. Book a hotel with a gym and use it. Over the years, I've learned that more often than not, business dinners go hand in hand with business travel. Therefore, your best bet is to wake up early and get your exercise in before your first meeting. If you absolutely can't find time to exercise during your trip, do more cardio before you leave and after you get back to make up the minutes so you still hit your weekly goal.

3) Use Your Splurge Meals Strategically. You have two meals a week to eat whatever you want. If you save them both for your business trip, you'll be OK if you can't control your food.

4) Bring Some Food Along With You. It's a great idea to bring some non-perishable food items along with you when you travel for a quick and healthy meal on the go. This works especially well for breakfast and lunch. For example, a low-fat mozzarella cheese stick, an apple, and some nuts can be a quick breakfast that will keep your blood sugar stable. Likewise, a tuna pouch, some nuts, and fruit make for a great lunch. All of these items travel well, can be eaten on the go (even on an airplane) and don't need to be refrigerated. Packing a few of these meals will help you avoid the carb crazy continental breakfasts at hotels or a fast food lunch.

5) When Eating Out, Follow The Strategies Listed In The Last Chapter. In the last FAQ, we went over some great strategies to help you stay on course while eating at restaurants. Get to know these strategies, and bring them on the road with you when traveling.

Do you have any tips on sugar free living?

As previously mentioned, sugar is an absolute disaster for those trying to lose weight and improve their health. It is highly addictive. The more you eat it, the more you want it. Sugar increases hunger and food cravings. It has also been associated with a number of chronic diseases. The best way to handle sugar is to eliminate it from your diet. Even tiny amounts of sugar can cause tremendous cravings for most of us. It seems strange saying this, but it is far easier to give up sugar 100% than to give it up 75%.

The overwhelming majority of my clients that have hit their goal weight have sworn off sugar. I, personally, have not touched sugar for over 20 years. I know this sounds intimidating. The idea of giving up sugar initially terrified me.

However, it is not nearly as difficult as you might think. If you are following this blood sugar stabilizing diet, your cravings for sugar virtually disappear after about 2 weeks. I've learned that cravings for sugar are much more physiological than psychological. Get it out of your diet, get through two weeks of withdrawal, and your desire for sugar will diminish to a level you never thought possible. Furthermore, sugar free versions of just about every dessert imaginable are now widely available.

As I mentioned earlier, I do not recommend non-nutritive sweeteners for everyday use. However, used occasionally, I believe that they are far less harmful than sugar. In fact, a recently published 28-year study with over 100,000 subjects from Harvard's Nurses' Health Study and Health Professional Follow-up Study found that substituting one diet soda per day for one sugar sweetened beverage significantly reduced total mortality, cardiovascular mortality and cancer mortality (1).

Since you are allowed two splurge meals per week, this is the time you are permitted to dive into the world of non-nutritive sweeteners. Limiting non-nutritive sweetener consumption to these two meals gives you the best of both worlds. You can enjoy something sweet a couple of times per week to satisfy your cravings for dessert, but you can also ensure a stable blood sugar to keep food cravings from getting out of control.

One more note, dairy products have a naturally occurring sugar called lactose. This is a low glycemic sugar that is easy on blood glucose and not a problem. However, because of this, dairy products like ice cream won't say sugar free on the package but will say "No Sugar Added". For the most part, these two terms are interchangeable.

Over the years, and with help from my clients, I have discovered some really good sugar free products to enjoy on splurge meals. Here's a list of the best of the best. Some are really easy to find and some you will have to order online. Remember—don't go overboard with the sugar free stuff. You can only have these sugar free treats twice per week with your splurge meals.

Edy's No Sugar Added Ice Cream: Most grocery store chains carry this in their freezer section. It comes in a bunch of great flavors, including Triple Chocolate, Mint Chip, Fudge Tracks, Neapolitan, and Vanilla. Turkey Hill, Blue Bunny, and Breyer's also make no sugar added ice cream that is really good.

Murray's Sugar Free Cookies: These are the best sugar free cookies that I've found by far. You can usually find these in your grocery store. If not, you can order them on Amazon.com. They have an amazing selection, including: Chocolate Chip, Oatmeal, Peanut Butter, Fudge Dipped Mint, Fudge Dipped Grahams, Sandwich Cookies, and more.

Klondike No Sugar Added Ice Cream Bars: These are outstanding and can usually be found in your grocery store's freezer section. They come in two different varieties, Vanilla and Crunch. I strongly recommend the Crunch.

Stop And Shop Brand No Sugar Added Ice Cream Sandwiches: Exclusive to Stop And Shop supermarkets. These are unbelievably good.

Hershey's Sugar Free Chocolates: These are usually available in the chain pharmacies like CVS, Rite Aid, and Walgreens. They come in Special Dark or Milk Chocolate. Stick with small quantities because these are very high in sugar alcohols which can have a laxative effect in sensitive individuals.

Reeses' Sugar Free Miniature Peanut Butter Cups: These can be found in pharmacies like CVS, Rite Aid, and Walgreens. They are very good. Stick with small quantities because they are high in sugar alcohols.

Sugar Free York Peppermint Patties: Also found in pharmacies. Also high in sugar alcohols, so limit amounts here.

Russell Stover Sugar Free Candy: You can find this amazing selection of candy in most pharmacies. They make Mint Patties, Crispy Caramel, Pecan Delights, Peanut Butter Crunch, Chocolate Coconut, Chocolate Covered Peanuts, and many more. Again, these are high in sugar alcohols so limit amounts. If you can't find these in stores, you can always get them online at www.russellstover.com.

Voortman's Sugar Free Cookies: These are terrific. They come in great flavors like Chocolate Chip, Oatmeal, and Vanilla Wafers. You can usually find these in your supermarket cookie section.

Sugar Free Jello And Chocolate Pudding: Sugar free Jello and Chocolate Pudding can be found in just about any supermarket. A spoonful of Sugar Free Cool Whip on top takes this to a whole new level.

Pure Protein Bars: There are energy bars that are high in protein and have very little sugar (usually just 2 grams in the entire bar). They are great for a meal replacement on an airplane or in between meetings. They come in a ton of great flavors and can be found at most supermarkets and pharmacies.

Pillsbury Sugar Free Brownie Mix: These come in Milk Chocolate and Chocolate Fudge flavors. They are really good and can be found in most supermarkets. Go easy with the portions here as these are quite high in sugar alcohols.

Pillsbury Sugar Free Cake Mix: This comes in Vanilla or Chocolate flavor and can be found in most grocery store bakery aisles. They also sell a sugar free frosting, which is really good. Go easy with the portions here as these are quite high in sugar alcohols.

Sugar Free Pancake Syrup: Great for a breakfast splurge of pancakes or French toast. Log Cabin makes one, and so does Cary's. Both taste great, in fact, I can't tell the difference between these and regular syrup. You can almost always find these in grocery stores. Many restaurants serving breakfast now carry these, so don't be afraid to ask for them.

DaVinci Sugar Free Syrups: These are awesome if you like to make flavored Lattes. They come in a lot of great flavors like Caramel, Chocolate, French Vanilla, Hazel Nut and many more. You can find these online at www.davincigourmet.com or amazon.com.

Sugar Free Cool Whip: Great on fresh fruit or sugar free ice cream. You can find this in most any grocery store.

Swiss Miss No Sugar Added Hot Chocolate: Delicious and found in most grocery stores.

Smucker's Sugar Free Grape Jelly: Really good and found in most grocery stores. This is high in sugar alcohol, so go easy on portions with this one. You can also find these online at www.smuckers.com.

Smucker's Sugar Free Hot Fudge: Found in grocery stores or online at www.smuckers.com. Great on sugar free ice cream. Also comes in caramel flavor. High in sugar alcohols so go easy on the portions.

Cheesecake Factory Low Carb Cheesecake: This just may be the best sugar free dessert that I have ever tried. Found at the Cheesecake Factory restaurants (they also do take out). It comes with sugar free whipped cream and strawberries. Make this a very occasional treat because it is very high in saturated fat and calories.

There you have it. These should hold you for a while! Remember, sugar free treats are only for your two splurge meals. The rest of the time you need to avoid non-nutritive sweeteners. The good news is that once your blood sugar stabilizes, you won't really even crave them.

Does anything change about the program once I hit my goal weight?

If you have hit your goal weight, congratulations on your hard work and dedication! Needing to come up with a weight loss maintenance program is a great problem to have. It is important to realize that this is not a temporary weight loss diet or exercise plan. These changes really do need to become a way of life going forward. Having said that, once you have hit your goal weight, you are not going to have to be quite as strict with the program.

Maintenance of weight lost is highly subjective; it will be different for each person. However, I do have several guidelines for my clients that have hit their goal weight:

-Continue with your weight training at least twice a week in order to maintain and add to your muscle mass.

-Feel free to add another small splurge meal to your week.

-Your cardiovascular exercise program may need some adjustment as well. Many of my clients continue with the amount of cardio they were doing during the weight loss phase. For others, if they do so, their weight will drop too low. For these clients, I recommend cutting back just a bit on the cardio.

Generally, weight maintenance is going to be trial and error. Weigh yourself weekly during maintenance the same way you did during the weight loss phase. If you notice you have gained a pound or 2 back, adjust your cardio or diet to strike that perfect balance. By the time one of my clients hits the point of maintenance, they have a really good grasp of the program and how to make it work for them. The good news is that by the time you get to this point, it is all under your control. You know exactly what to do to lose weight.

SUMMARY

1- Combine a healthy source of fat, protein and carbohydrate at each and every meal.
2- Complete the required number of cardio minutes at the proper intensity. The average number for women is 250 minutes a week and for men it is 150 minutes per week.
3- Complete at least 2 sessions of resistance training each week in order to maintain and even add to your metabolically active lean body mass.
4- Keep a log of your diet and cardio minutes.
5- No eating after 8:00 PM.
6- If you drink, limit alcoholic beverages to 4 per week, at least until you hit your goal weight.
7- Drink 8 glasses of water per day.
8- Sleep at least 7 hours each night.
9- Completely avoid sugar.
10- Feel free to take 2 splurge meals a week to keep you honest over the long-term. While you want to limit non-nutritive sweetener use, feel free to enjoy a few sugar free treats with your cheat meals.

Final Thoughts

I know that I have thrown an awful lot at you in these last several hundred pages. Making positive changes to your diet and exercise program is exciting, challenging and even a little bit scary. However, never underestimate the degree to which making these changes can improve your life.

Feeling good physically and mentally is the absolute foundation of your life. It makes you a better worker, student, spouse, parent, friend... what I am trying to say is that it will make you a better person. I can say, unequivocally, that any effort you put into this program is well worth the investment. The rewards are great.

In our journey, you have learned the importance of resistance training and how to get started on a good program. You have gathered all the information you will need to design a cardiovascular exercise routine that will help you attain your weight loss goals and improve your life and health in many ways.

You have learned how very important it is to eat in a way that promotes a stable blood sugar. You now have all the tools to do this, no matter what life throws at you. Lastly, you have learned that lifestyle factors are the icing on the cake, no pun intended, when it comes to hitting your weight loss goals.

I have found that people who struggle with their weight generally fall into two categories: Those who don't know what to do and those who do know what to do, but don't do it. You now know exactly what to do. There are no more excuses, no more reasons to procrastinate. Get started today.

Be kind to yourself. When you have setbacks along the way, don't beat yourself up. Just try to do the best that you can. You can learn the principles of this program in just a couple of days, but to incorporate them into your life can take months and sometimes, even years. That is OK, because as you are getting better at following these principles, you will be losing weight, improving your health and improving your quality of life all along the way.

Always keep in mind that these changes are not "all or nothing". If you can accomplish even half of these recommendations, you will lose a lot of weight and your quality of life and health will improve tremendously. I always tell my clients to try to get a little bit better each week in an area that is giving them difficulty. If you only hit 75 minutes of cardio this week, shoot for 80 next week. If you had 5 splurge meals this week, shoot for 4 next week. Slow and steady wins the race. The goal is progress, not perfection.

It means a lot to me that you have taken the time out of your busy schedule to read *The Weight Loss Triad*. Thank you for that. I wish you the very best of good luck as you begin your journey toward a healthier life. It is so very worth the effort. If I can be of any assistance to you along the way, please don't hesitate to contact me at www.drtomhalton.com.

Here's to your good health,

Thomas L. Halton

References

Chapter 2

1) Foster-Powell K, et al. International table of glycemic index and glycemic load values: 2002. *American Journal of Clinical Nutrition* 2002; 76:5-56.

2) Bao j, et al. Food insulin index: physiologic basis for predicting insulin demand evoked by composite meals. *American Journal of Clinical Nutrition* 2009; 90:986-92.

3) Ludwig DS. Dietary glycemic index and obesity. *Journal of Nutrition* 2000; 130:280S-283S.

4) Lennerz BS. Effects of dietary glycemic index on brain regions related to reward and craving in men. *American Journal of Clinical Nutrition* 2013; 98:641-47.

5) Ludwig DS. The glycemic index: Physiological mechanisms relating to obesity, diabetes and cardiovascular disease. *Journal of the American Medical Association* 2002; 287:2414-23.

6) Sigal RJ et al. Acute postchallenge hyperinsulinemia predicts weight gain: A prospective study. *Diabetes* 1997; 46:1025-29.

7) Mozaffarian D, et al. Changes in diet and lifestyle and long-term weight gain in women and men. *New England Journal of Medicine* 2011; 364:2392-404.

8) Jeya C, et al. The influence of adding fats of varying saturation on the glycemic response of white bread.

International Journal of Food Sciences and Nutrition 2008;59:61-69.

9) Meng H, et al. Effects of macronutrients and fiber on postprandial glycemic responses and meal glycemic index and glycemic load value determinations. *American Journal of Clinical Nutrition* 2017; 105:842-53.

10) Sun L, et al. Effect of chicken, fat and vegetable on glycemia and insulinemia to a white rice based meal in healthy adults. *European Journal of Nutrition* 2014; 53:1719-26.

Chapter 3
1) Poppitt SD, et al. Short-term effects of macronutrient preloads on appetite and energy intake in lean women. *Physiology and Behavior* 1998: 64;279-285.

2) Stubbs RJ, et al. Description and evaluation of an experimental model to examine changes in selection between high protein, high carbohydrate and high fat foods in humans. *European Journal of Clinical Nutrition* 1999: 53;13-21.

3) Porrini N, et al. Evaluation of satiety sensations and food intake after different preloads. *Appetite* 1995; 25:17-30.

4) Barkeling B, et al. Effects of a high protein meal and a high carbohydrate meal on satiety measured by automated computer monitoring of subsequent food intake, motivation to eat and food preferences. *International Journal of Obesity* 1990; 14:743-51.

5) Halton TL, et al. The effects of high protein diets on thermogenesis, satiety and weight loss: A critical review. *Journal of the American College of Nutrition* 2004; 23:373-85.

6) Bernstein AM, et al. Major dietary protein sources and risk of coronary heart disease in women. *Circulation* 2010; 122: 876-83.

7) Pan A, et al. Red meat consumption and mortality: Results from 2 prospective cohort studies. *Archives of Internal Medicine* 2012; 172:555-63.

8) Pan A, et al. Red meat consumption and risk of type 2 diabetes: 3 cohorts of U.S. adults and an updated meta-analysis. *American Journal of Clinical Nutrition* 2011; 94:1088-96.

9) Bouvard V, et al. Carcinogenicity of consumption of red and processed meat. *The Lancet Oncology* 2015; 16:1599-1600.

10) Appel LJ, et al. Effects of protein, monounsaturated fat and carbohydrate intake on blood pressure and serum lipids: Results of the OmniHeart randomized trial. *Journal of the American Medical Association* 2005; 294:2455-64.

11) Halton TL, et al. Low carbohydrate diet score and risk of coronary heart disease in women. *New England Journal of Medicine* 2006; 355:1991-2002.

12) Halton TL, et al. Low carbohydrate diet score and risk of type 2 diabetes in women. *American Journal of Clinical Nutrition* 2008; 87:339-46.

13) Feskanich D, et al. Protein consumption and bone fractures in women. *American Journal of Epidemiology* 1996; 143:472-79.

14) Gardner CD, et al. Comparison of the Atkins, Zone, Ornish and LEARN diets for change in weight and related risk factors among overweight premenopausal women: The A to Z weight loss study. *Journal of the American Medical Association* 2007; 297:969-77.

15) Bischoff-Ferrari HA, et al. Calcium intake and hip fracture in men and women: a meta-analysis of prospective cohort studies and randomized controlled trials. *American Journal of Clinical Nutrition* 2007; 86:1780-90.

16) Giovannucci E, et al. Risk factors for prostate cancer incidence and progression in the Health Professional Follow-up Study. *International Journal of Cancer* 2007; 121:1571-78.

17) Genkinger JM, et al. Dairy products and ovarian cancer: A pooled analysis of 12 cohort studies. *Cancer Epidemiology, Biomarkers and Prevention* 2006; 15:364-72.

Chapter 4
1) Vesper HW, et al. Levels of plasma trans-fatty acids in non-Hispanic white adults in the United States in 2000

and 2009. *Journal of the American Medical Association* 2012; 307:562-63.

2) Wang, DD et al. Association of specific dietary fats with total and cause specific mortality. *JAMA Internal Medicine* 2016; 176:1134-45.

3) Hu FB, et al. Dietary fat intake and risk of coronary heart disease in women. *New England Journal of Medicine* 1997; 337:1491-99.

4) Estruch R, et al. Primary prevention of cardiovascular disease with a Mediterranean diet. *New England Journal of Medicine* 2013; 368:1279-90.

5) Appel LJ, et al. Effect of protein, monounsaturated fat and carbohydrate intake on blood pressure and serum lipids: Results of the OmniHeart Randomized Trial. *Journal of the American Medical Association* 2005; 294:2455-2464.

6) de Lorgeril M, et al. Mediterranean alpha-linolenic acid rich diet in secondary prevention of coronary heart disease. *The Lancet* 1994; 343:1454-59.

7) Mensink RP, et al. Effects of dietary fatty acids and carbohydrates on the ratio of serum total to HDL cholesterol and on serum lipids and apolipoproteins: A meta-analysis of 60 controlled trials. *American Journal of Clinical Nutrition* 2003; 77:1146-55.

8) Salmeron J, et al. Dietary fat intake and risk of type 2 diabetes in women. *American Journal of Clinical Nutrition* 2001; 73:1019-26.

9) Cho E, et al. Premenopausal fat intake and risk of breast cancer. *Journal of the National Cancer Institute* 2003; 95:1079-85.

10) Hu FB et al. Fish and omega-3 fatty acid intake and risk of coronary heart disease in women. *Journal of the American Medical Association* 2002; 287:1815-21.

11) Iso H, et al. Intake of fish and omega-3 fatty acids and risk of stroke in women. *Journal of the American Medical Association* 2001; 285:304-12.

12) Mozzaffarian D, et al. Plasma phospholipid long chain omega-3 fatty acids and total and cause specific mortality in older adults: The Cardiovascular Health Study. *Annals of Internal Medicine* 2013; 158:515-25.

13) Hu FB, et al. Frequent nut consumption and risk of coronary heart disease in women: prospective cohort study. *British Medical Journal* 1998; 317:1341-45.

14) Jiang R, et al. Nut and peanut butter consumption and risk of type 2 diabetes in women. *Journal of the American Medical Association* 2002; 288:2554-60.

Chapter 5
1) Willett WC, Skerritt PJ. Eat Drink And Be Healthy. New York, NY. Free Press Publishing 2017: page 110.

2) Ludwig DS. The glycemic index: Physiological mechanisms relating to obesity, diabetes and cardiovascular disease. *Journal of the American Medical Association* 2002; 287:2414-23.

3) Jenkins DJ, et al. Glycemic index of food: A physiological basis for carbohydrate exchange. *American Journal of Clinical Nutrition* 1981; 34:362-66.

4) Halton TL. Maximize Your Health. Boston, MA. Fitness Plus Publishing 2012: pages 103-107.

5) Halton TL, et al. Low carbohydrate diet score and risk of coronary heart disease in women. *New England Journal of Medicine* 2006; 355:1991-2002.

6) Beulens JW, et al. High dietary glycemic load and glycemic index increases risk of cardiovascular disease among middle aged women. *Journal of the American Journal of Cardiology* 2007; 50:14-21.

7) Mirrahimi A, et al. Associations of glycemic index and load with coronary heart disease events: A systematic review and meta-analysis of prospective cohorts. *Journal of the American Heart Association* 2012; 1:e000752.

8) Halton TL, et al. Low carbohydrate diet score and risk of type 2 diabetes in women. *American Journal of Clinical Nutrition* 2008; 87:339-46.

9) Bhupathiraju SN, et al. Glycemic index, glycemic load and risk of type 2 diabetes: Results from 3 large U.S. cohorts and an updated meta-analysis. *American Journal of Clinical Nutrition* 2014; 100:218-32.

10) Oh K, et al. Carbohydrate intake, glycemic index, glycemic load and dietary fiber in relation to risk of stroke in women. *American Journal of Epidemiology* 2005; 161:161-69.

11) Higginbotham S, et al. Dietary glycemic load and risk of colorectal cancer in the Women's Health Study. *Journal of the National Cancer Institute* 2004; 96:229-33.

12) Ludwig DS, et al. High glycemic index foods, overeating and obesity. *Pediatrics* 1999; 103:E26.

13) Mozaffarian D, et al. Changes in diet and lifestyle and long-term weight gain in women and men. *New England Journal of Medicine* 2011; 364:2392-404.

14) Lennerz BS, et al. Effects of dietary glycemic index on brain regions related to reward and craving in men. *American Journal of Clinical Nutrition* 2013; 98:641-47.

15) Ebbeling CB, et al. Effects of a low glycemic load vs low fat diet in obese young adults. *Journal of the American Medical Association* 2007; 297:2092-2102.

16) Slabber M, et al. Effects of a low insulin response, energy restricted diet on weight loss and plasma insulin concentrations in hyperinsulinemic obese females. *American Journal of Clinical Nutrition* 1994; 60:48-53.

17) Bouce C, et al. Five week, low glycemic index diet decreases total fat mass and improves plasma lipid

profile in moderately overweight nondiabetic men. *Diabetes Care* 2002; 25:822-28.

18) Spieth LE, et al. A low glycemic index diet in the treatment of pediatric obesity. *Archives of Pediatric and Adolescent Medicine* 2000; 154:947-51.

Chapter 7
1) Treuth MS, et al. Effect of exercise intensity on 24-hour energy expenditure and substrate oxidation. *Medicine and Science in Sports and Exercise* 1996; 28:1138-43.

2) Van Pelt RE, et al. Regular exercise and the age-related decline in resting metabolic rate in women. *Journal of Clinical Endocrinology and Metabolism* 1997; 82:3208-12.

3) Wing RR, et al. Long-term weight loss maintenance. *American Journal of Clinical Nutrition* 2005; 82 (Supplement):222s-5s.

4) Lee IM, et al. Physical activity and weight gain prevention. *Journal of the American Medical Association* 2010; 303:1173-79.

5) Mekary RA, et al. Physical activity patterns and prevention of weight gain in premenopausal women. *International Journal of Obesity* 2009; 33:1039-47.

6) Fogelholm M, et al. Effects of walking training on weight maintenance after a very low energy diet in obese pre-menopausal women: A randomized controlled trial. *Archives of Internal Medicine* 2000; 160:2177-84.

7) Mekary RA, et al. Physical activity in relation to long-term weight maintenance after intentional weight loss in pre-menopausal women. *Obesity* 2009; 18:167-74.

8) Li TY, et al. Obesity as compared with physical activity in predicting risk of coronary heart disease in women. *Circulation* 2006; 113:499-506.

9) Hu FB, et al. Physical activity and risk of stroke in women. *Journal of the American Medical Association* 2000; 283:2961-67.

10) Hu FB, et al. Physical activity and television watching in relation to risk for type 2 diabetes mellitus in men. *Archives of Internal Medicine* 2001; 161:1542-48.

11) Giovannucci E, et al. Physical activity, obesity, and risk for colon cancer and adenoma in men. *Annals of Internal Medicine* 1995; 122:327-334.

12) Rockhill B, et al. A prospective study of recreational physical activity and breast cancer risk. *Archives of Internal Medicine* 1999; 159:2290-2296.

13) Weuve J, et al. Physical activity, including walking, and cognitive function in older women. *Journal of the American Medical Association* 2004; 292:1454-61.

14) Wei M, et al. Relationship between low cardio-respiratory fitness and mortality in normal weight, overweight, and obese men. *Journal of the American Medical Association* 1999; 282:1547-1553.

15) Hu FB, et al. Adiposity as compared with physical activity in predicting mortality among women. *New England Journal of Medicine* 2004; 351:2694-2703.

16) Centers for disease control and prevention. National Center for Health Statistics: Exercise or physical activity. Accessed on 2/10/20 www.cdc.gov/nchs/fastats/exercise.htm

Chapter 8
1) Marcell TJ. Sarcopenia: Causes, consequences and preventions. *Journal of Gerontology* 2003; 58a:911-916.

2) Wang Z, et al. Resting energy expenditure: Systematic organization and critique of prediction methods. *Obesity Research* 2001; 9:331-36.

3) Hunter GR, et al. Resistance training conserves fat free mass and resting energy expenditure following weight loss. *Obesity* 2008; 16:1045-51.

4) Ballor DL et al. Resistance weight training during caloric restriction enhances lean body weight maintenance. *American Journal of Clinical Nutrition* 1988; 47:19-25.

5) Geliebter A, et al. Effects of strength or aerobic training on body composition, resting metabolic rate, and peak oxygen consumption in obese dieting subjects. *American Journal of Clinical Nutrition* 1997; 66:557-63.

Chapter 10
1) McHill AW, et al. Later circadian timing of food intake is associated with increased body fat. *American Journal of Clinical Nutrition* 2017; 106:1213-19.

2) Baron KG, et al. Contribution of evening macronutrient intake to total caloric intake and body mass index. *Appetite* 2013; 60:246-51.

3) Romon M, et al. Circadian variation of diet induced thermogenesis. *American Journal of Clinical Nutrition* 1993; 57:476-80.

4) Pan A et al. Changes in water and beverage intake and long-term weight changes: results from 3 prospective cohort studies. *International Journal of Obesity* 2013; 37:1378-85.

5) Dennis EA, et al. Water consumption increases weight loss during a hypocaloric diet intervention in middle aged and older adults. *Obesity* 2010; 18:300-307.

6) Stookey JD, et al. Drinking water is associated with weight loss in overweight dieting women independent of diet and activity. *Obesity* 2008; 16:2481-88.

7) Boschmann M, et al. Water induced thermogenesis. *Journal of Clinical Endocrinology and Metabolism* 2003; 88:6015-19.

8) Boschmann M, et al. Water drinking induces thermogenesis through osmosensitive mechanisms. *Journal of Clinical Endocrinology and Metabolism* 2007; 92:3334-37.

9) Van Wallenghen EL, et al. Pre-meal water consumption reduces meal energy intake in older but not younger subjects. *Obesity* 2007; 15:93-99.

10) Mozaffarian D, et al. Changes in diet and lifestyle and long-term weight gain in women and men. *New England Journal of Medicine* 2011; 364:2392-404.

11) Sayon-Orea C, et al. Alcohol consumption and body weight: A systematic review. *Nutrition Reviews* 2011; 69:419-31.

12) Wannamethee SG, et al. Alcohol intake and 8-year weight gain in women: A prospective study. *Obesity Research* 2004; 12:1386-96.

13) Downer MK, et al. Change in alcohol intake in relation to weight change in a cohort of United States men with 24 years of follow-up. *Obesity* 2017; 25:1988-96.

14) Breslow RA, et al. Diets of drinkers on drinking and non-drinking days: NHANES 2003-2008. *American Journal of Clinical Nutrition* 2013; 97:1068-75.

15) Pan A, et al. Changes in water and beverage intake and long-term weight changes: results from 3 prospective studies. *International Journal of Obesity* 2013; 37:1378-85.

16) Fung TT, et al. Sweetened beverage consumption and risk of coronary heart disease in women. *American Journal of Clinical Nutrition* 2009; 89:1037-42.

17) de Koning L, et al. Sugar sweetened and artificially sweetened beverage consumption and risk of type 2 diabetes in men. *American Journal of Clinical Nutrition* 2011; 93:1321-27.

18) Bernstein AM, et al. Soda consumption and risk of stroke in men and women. *American Journal of Clinical Nutrition* 2012; 95:1190-99.

19) Marinovich M, et al. Aspartame, low calorie sweeteners and disease: Regulatory safety and epidemiological issues. *Food and Chemical Toxicology* 2013; 60:109-115.

20) Meyer-Gerspach AC, et al. Effects of caloric and noncaloric sweeteners on antroduodenal motility, gastrointestinal hormone secretion and appetite related sensations in healthy subjects. *American Journal of Clinical Nutrition* 2018; 107: 707-16.

21) Frank GKW, et al. Sucrose activates human taste pathways differently from artificial sweetener. *Neuroimage* 2008; 39:1559-1569.

22) Romo-Romo A, et al. Sucralose decreases insulin sensitivity in healthy subjects: a randomized controlled trial. *American Journal of Clinical Nutrition* 2018; 108:485-91.

23) Patel SR, et al. Association between reduced sleep and weight gain in women. *American Journal of Epidemiology* 2006; 164:947-54.

24) St-Onge MP, et al. Short sleep duration increases energy intakes but does not change energy expenditure in normal weight individuals. *American Journal of Clinical Nutrition* 2011; 94:410-16.

25) Benedict C, et al. Acute sleep deprivation reduces energy expenditure in healthy men. *American Journal of Clinical Nutrition* 2011; 93:1229-36.

26) Al Khatib HK, et al. Sleep extension is a feasible lifestyle intervention in free living adults who are habitually short sleepers: A potential strategy for decreasing intake of free sugars? A randomized controlled pilot study. *American Journal of Clinical Nutrition* 2018; 107:43-53.

Chapter 11
1) Malik VS et al, Long term consumption of sugar sweetened and artificially sweetened beverages and risk of mortality in US adults. *Circulation* 2019; 139:2113-25.

Also By Dr. Thomas L. Halton:

Life On The Triad
Meal Plan And Recipe Companion To The
Weight Loss Triad

Maximize Your Health
The Top Ten Research Proven Strategies To
Reduce Your Risk Of Chronic Disease

The Weight Loss Triad
A Comprehensive Guide To Lasting Weight
Loss

If you need more guidance, Dr. Halton is
available for phone consultations. Learn more at:
www.drtomhalton.com/phone-coaching

Dr. Halton also publishes a free e-newsletter.
Learn more and sign-up at:
www.drtomhalton.com/newsletter